MAIDEN TO MOTHER

MAIDEN TO MOTHER

RESTORING THE SPIRITUAL WISDOM OF
PREGNANCY, BIRTH AND MOTHERHOOD AS A
SACRED RITE OF PASSAGE.

DONNA RAYMOND

Maiden to Mother: Restoring the Spiritual Wisdom of Pregnancy, Birth and Motherhood as a Sacred Rite of Passage.

Copyright © 2024 by Donna Raymond

All rights reserved. No part of this publication may be reproduced, stored in a retrieval system, or transmitted in any form or by any means, electronic, mechanical, photocopying, recording or otherwise, without the prior written permission from both the copyright owner and publisher, except for the use of brief quotations in a book review.

Disclaimer

All the information, techniques, skills and concepts contained within this publication are of the nature of general comment only and are not in any way recommended as individual advice. The intent is to offer a variety of information to provide a wider range of choices now and in the future, recognising that we all have widely diverse circumstances and viewpoints. Should any reader choose to use the information contained herein, this is their decision and the author and publishers do not assume any responsibilities whatsoever under any condition or circumstances. AI software has been used for editing purposes.

Cover design: Donna Raymond

Photography: Chanel Baran

Editing: Donna Hakanson

ISBN: 9780645096828

Visit: www.DonnaRaymond.com.au

I sit in stillness. The stirring, collective wisdom of Herstory echoes through my heart and whispers on the summer wind. The land speaks loudly as the Grandmothers sing through ancient songlines, to reach me in the in-between realms.

In this liminal moment, my womb is ripe with creation, carrying my first son. He calls me into presence. I am open. I am here now, listening deeply.

Embodying the intent to connect with the primal wisdom that echoes through my Soul, I transcribe the mystical experiences of the sacred initiation from Maiden to Mother and deepening further into Motherhood. Spirit guides me to birth this book with grace that speaks to the eloquence and profound beauty of creation and the power of **Wombman.**

I offer this book as a map of soulful resonance to help guide Mothers through the primal wild. A sacred transmission for those called to receive it, in reverence and honour of all birthing Mothers that have walked before us.

May we continue to activate our ancient remembering

and restore the primordial birth codes for the generations of daughters yet to be initiated.

Together we birth a new paradigm of love, beauty, connection and power.

One Maiden, one Mother, at a time.

-Donna Raymond
December 6, 2018

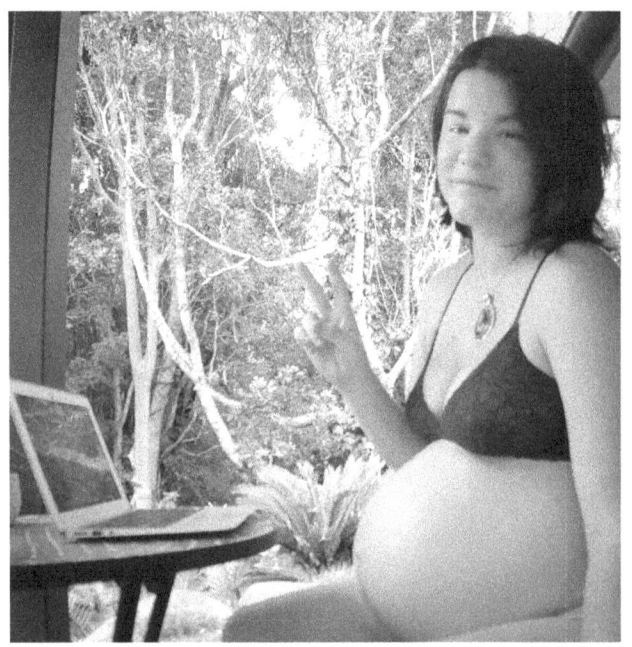

*35 weeks pregnant with Zenith
when I started writing this book.*

CONTENTS

Foreword Jane Hardwicke Collings	xiii
Preface	xvii
Acknowledgments	xxi
Introduction	xxiii
Part I- Sacred Women's Business *Honoring the Divine Feminine and Reclaiming Birth as Sacred*	1
1. HerStory *Attuning to the wisdom of the Women's Mysteries*	3
2. Rotten Roots *The Parasitic Nature of Patriarchal Birth*	19
3. Ripples of Love *The Impact of Birth Experiences*	33
4. Sacred Rites of Passage *Understanding Birth as a Process of Initiation*	47
5. Maiden to Mother *The Great Initiation*	53
Part II- Preparation *Nurturing the Spiritual Connection During Pregnancy*	67
6. Conception *Conscious Co-Creation*	69
7. Sacred Pregnancy *Mystical Maternity and Activating the Womb Grid*	79
8. Nourishing the Journey *Embracing Whole Body Nutrition*	97
9. Birth Warrior *Overcoming Fear and Worry*	111
10. The Power of Ceremony *Weaving Meaning and Purpose*	129
Part III- The Primal Wild *Navigating the Spiritual Dimesions of Labour and Birth*	141
11. Prepare to Birth *Activating the Birth Spiral*	143
12. The Sacred Spiral *The Eternal Dance of Birth and Death*	161
13. The Language of Birth *Navigating the Initiation of Birth and the Primal Wild*	173
14. Practical Birthing Wisdom *Remember to Breathe and Relax Your Jaw!*	191

Part IV- Sacred Postpartum 199
Crossing the Threshold of Maiden to Mother

15. Mother 201
    A new World is Born
16. Rooted in Wisdom 213
    Embracing Indigenous Traditions
17. Womb Healing 223
    Nurturing Body and Spirit Postpartum
18. The Art of Breastfeeding 239
    A Journey of Nourishment, Wisdom and Transition

Part V: The Great Work 255
Embracing and Deepening into the legacy of your Motherhood

19. Matresence 257
    The Sacred Dance of Becoming
20. The Abyss of Motherhood 265
    Illuminating the Path through the Darkness of the first years.
21. Reparenting yourself 281
    Heal Your inner Child and Break Cycles
22. Revival of the Village 293
    De-Urbanising Motherhood and Rekindling Resilience

Part VI Sacred Birth Stories 301
My Journeys into the Primal Wild

23. My Maiden to Mother Journey 303
    Auraura's Birth Story
24. The Birth Shaman 313
    Maia Lily's Free Birth Story
25. A Very Homely Freebirth 323
    Lucah's Birth Story
26. From A to Z 331
    Zenith's birth story.
27. Charlotte 345
    My Abortion Story

Notes 353
Values List 357
About the Author 361

∼

To my womb-fruits

*You have shown me the greatest depths of the Great Mystery
and I am forever blessed to be your Mother.
Thank you for choosing to journey with me.
For all that you are and continue to be,
I love you.
All ways, always.*

∼

FOREWORD

JANE HARDWICKE COLLINGS

Imagine a world where we feel safe and respected, held and heard and where our rites of passage are honoured and celebrated because everyone knows how important that is.

In this ideal world, we navigate *Adolescence*, our menarche, the menstrual cycle, and our contraceptive needs in a prepared, supported and beautiful way. Then, as we conceive, gestate and give birth, we enter *Matrescence* and are held and supported by our village. Finally, when we transition into *Sagescence* during perimenopause and beyond, we are honoured and valued as the wise women of our community.

Sadly, this is not the case. Our rites of passage have been forgotten and ignored. Yet, they occur whether we consciously acknowledge or honour them, leaving a lasting imprint. Whatever happens during a rite of passage—who is present, what is said or left unsaid, and the context surrounding the event—teaches the woman on a subliminal level. This subtle teaching, or enculturation, shapes her understanding of her role within the culture and informs her how to behave to be accepted by the culture.

Every rite of passage functions in this way.

Consider the rite of menarche, the first menstruation. In most cultures, this transition is not honoured as a sacred initiation into womanhood. Instead, the absence of an empowering initiation subtly teaches girls that their culture does not value women. Sandra Ingerman, a shamanic teacher, observes that when women are not welcomed into womanhood in a conscious, empowering way, when they miss the transmission of ancestral knowledge and feminine power they experience feminine power *'soul loss'*. This creates a void, leaving many uninitiated Maidens to approach childbirth unprepared for the magnitude of this next transformation.

The way we are held during our Adolescence and menarche profoundly impacts our relationship with our menstrual cycle and body. Adolescence is a becoming, the journey to adulthood. Childbirth, then, becomes the next altar of transformation, ushering in the process of Matrescence, the becoming of a Mother, which is hugely affected by all that came before. Our transformative journey continues into menopause when we arrive at Sagescence and our wise woman years. One rite of passage leads to the next.

Childbirth and Matrescence are rites of passage that ripple beyond the individual. They shape not only the mother but also the baby, the family, the birth workers and future generations. As the saying goes, *"She who rocks the cradle rules the world."* A mother's navigation of conception, pregnancy, birth and postpartum influences the unfolding of life for generations to come.

Rites of passage both create and reinforce culture. They shape internal beliefs, attitudes and fears, as well as external societal norms. When most individuals experience similar rites of passage, the resulting mindsets perpetuate themselves. The good news is that rites of passage also offer an opportunity to 'hack' the culture and create change.

By nurturing girls during their menarche and Adolescence, we can foster positive attitudes toward the menstrual cycle and the body. Sharon Moloney's research has shown that such positive experiences reduce the likelihood of interventions and trauma during childbirth. And how we navigate Matrescence will show up in our mothering and at each following birth and eventually at our menopause.

We need to shift the focus from fear and risk during childbirth to the awareness for preparation which includes education and inner work.

This is also a process of reclamation and here is the guidebook - a way to navigate Maiden to Mother - Matrescence.

We must, individually and collectively, redefine pregnancy, birth and motherhood as sacred and hold motherhood and the process of Matrescence as our spiritual path. If we do this, we will unhook from the patriarchy and change the world.

Donna's book, *Maiden to Mother,* offers guidance through this transformative journey. Filled with personal stories, science, insights and practical suggestions, it reminds us of the significance of these experiences. As birthing women and as the communities and families who support them, we must recognise the profound importance of these rites of passage.

Together, we can honour and transform the journey from Maiden to Mother, reclaiming the power and wisdom that is our birthright.

We need to co-create and recreate this old/new worldview and Donna has provided a guidebook to change the world!

Blessed be, dear sister.

Jane Hardwicke Collings

Midwife, Women's Mysteries Teacher and Founder of the School of Shamanic Womancraft

PREFACE

∽

This book has been over 10 years in the making. However, I started writing on the cusp of birthing my fourth child as it felt pertinent to create the space necessary to share my wisdom, both experiential and from extensive personal research over the years.

When I became a mother for the first time, although I felt I had become a walking encyclopaedia concerning the physiological aspects of birth, I felt completely out of my depth with transitioning from *Maiden to Mother*, both emotionally and spiritually.

The truth is, I had no idea of the dark tint on those rose-coloured glasses I was wearing; twenty-one years young, pregnant, rebellious and naïve, totally unaware of what was to come.

Unfortunately, yet necessary for my journey, I had to trudge through some intense emotional sludge, fear and insecurities during my pregnancy, testing me in ways I could never have imagined. I was alone, though deep down, I knew I was connected to something bigger and was being initiated in a way that I was unaware of.

This deep sense of trust always connected me to the spiritual nature of birth. I may not have had the vocabulary or maturity to comprehend the scope of what I was intuitively tapping into, but I knew it in my bones.

My Maiden self walked into *the Great Mystery* in complete surrender, naively open-hearted and wide-eyed. Something deeply magical transpired around me and I felt guided the whole way, even through the dark times.

In 2007, during an intensely long labour, my midwife Gabrielle would check in to see how I was and the only communication I could share at the time was in the form of a nod and a whisper:

"Maiden to Mother... Maiden to Mother"

I was deep in it, and this was the language I knew intuitively before I knew about the *women's mysteries*. This is how she knew I was ok, deep in the process of birthing, exhausted, but ok. These words were my anchor as worlds collapsed around me. I completed the first phase of my initiation, birthing naturally and crossing the threshold into Motherhood with a beautiful daughter.

The first year was incredibly hard and emotionally draining. Anointed in shit, spew and a silent creeping loneliness, I felt isolated, disconnected, alone and afraid. I lost my creativity, my 'village', my relationship, my spark. I lost myself.

My identity as a free *Maiden* was sacrificed at the altar of my new role as *Mother*. In the following years, I delved deep into emotional alchemy practices, intuitive womb and shadow work and cleared up traumatic experiences from what felt like a crash landing into Motherhood. I began to realise the extent of how my unresolved emotion had impacted me, my birth, my baby, creativity, identity and the experience of Motherhood. Everything became clearer.

I've since freebirthed 3 children at home in Kuranda. My life is challenging, though I feel inspired, connected, wildly creative and joyful as a Mother, matriarch and mentor.

What I am about to share within the pages of this book is not only an honest account and reflection of my journey, but I am also going to shine a light into some dark spaces, to create a clear map and share with you some profound and potent wisdom that I accessed during the peak of birthing and raising my babies.

My biggest challenge in writing this book was creating the space to write and navigating the demands of little people with my drive to create. I am so grateful to be surrounded by a beautiful, supportive network of family and friends to make this happen. Thank you to everyone who has supported me on my journey, walking my Wise Wombman path.

Creating the *Maiden to Mother* e-course in 2016 *helped to develop the pathways to navigate writing and to focus on what was important and necessary to share because, let's face it, there are many amazing pregnancy and birth books out there. I'm not interested in creating more noise. So I simply listened to the whispers within and spoke to fill in the gaps.

I believe wholeheartedly that women have the power to change the world, and we can do so in one generation. Motherhood is *the* most profound spiritual journey, truly!

This is important for all new Mothers and those deepening into Motherhood. I have learned that pregnancy and birth can be beautiful, spiritual, empowering and liberating experiences when we allow ourselves to trust and remember our power as women. The journey of pregnancy and birth is one of maturation that initiates us into our power. It irrevocably alters and changes us inside out.

When we acknowledge the spiritual aspects of motherhood and tap into deep primal birthing wisdom, we are restoring the sacred codes of the womb. I am a testament to beautiful, peaceful and powerful births. I have walked this path and will continue to gather the women to weave new worlds of wonder.

Peace on Earth doesn't just begin with birth. It starts with the purposeful initiation from **Maiden to Mother.**

---

* www.donnaraymond.com.au/courses/maidentomother

ACKNOWLEDGMENTS

I have always believed that we never truly accomplish anything alone for we exist within a vast and intricate tapestry of connection, inspiration, intention and energy that weaves us together in community.

I am blessed to be surrounded by a circle of genuine, loving, inspiring and wildly creative souls, many of whom I'm honoured to call my sisters. With this in mind, I wish to express my deepest gratitude to the beautiful souls who have journeyed alongside me in bringing this book to life.

To my best friend, Chanel Baran, visionary photographer extraordinaire! Your exquisite images grace both the cover and the pages within. Choosing from the countless stunning photos you've taken of me over the years was no easy task, but each one weaves a visual soul into this work. I am grateful beyond words for your friendship, artistry and support and wish everyone could know how truly incredible, kind-hearted and lovely you are. (www.chanelbaran.com)

To Donni, you've been a guiding light on my writing journey. Your keen eye, thoughtful yellow highlights, humorous notes and feedback have been a treasure. You are the one person I've trusted with the rawness of my words, knowing you would hold them with care and help me refine them without judgment. Despite any setbacks, your commitment to working your majick on my manuscript has shown a deep level of support for which I am forever grateful.

And finally, to my family, thank you for your unwavering support as I laboured through the birth of this book. Sitting at the dinner table, sharing my progress and being cheered on for each milestone has filled my heart with gratitude to share my life and art with you all.

INTRODUCTION

~

I wrote this book to serve as a sanctuary to anchor my wisdom as I continue deepening into my season of Mother, amplifying the resonant narratives echoed by women I've connected with over the years. In my self-indulgence, it is offered as the second legacy book in a series for my daughters (and future generations) so that upon my death, they will have a map to navigate birth as the great initiation and sacred rite of passage, transitioning from *Maiden to Mother*.

This is not *just a book* about pregnancy and birth as a spiritual experience, it is a conduit, transmission and reclamation of the wild daughter within via the initiation and integration of both Maiden and Mother, calling forth the sisters of revolution and rebirth.

We are on the precipice of profound change and it is the responsibility of us, as women and custodians of the future, to attune our minds, hearts and wombs to sculpt the future we are ushering forth.

I've written this book in parts that make up the whole picture. Start with the first part as foundational wisdom and then bounce around as you see fit. This information is not just for Maidens. The wisdom contained in this book is timeless and can help women as they spiral deeper into Motherhood; with each new baby or project, a new aspect of yourself and your gifts are born, the mystery is revived and you circle back around.

I intend to help women become emotionally and spiritually prepared for the journey ahead and approach Motherhood as an initiation that builds resilience and wonder. I want to see a world where women are supported in all ways as they step into the unknown and birth themselves and their babies with beauty and grace, knowing that all pregnancies result in a birth, no matter the outcome and this is to be honoured.

Please share this book with those yearning to wake up from the collective slumber and become fluent in the primordial power and language of birth as a way to breathe themselves more fully into the presence, power and creativity of a Mother.

In the grand tapestry of life, my lived experiences are but fleeting stitches in the fabric of time and this book stands as the loom that weaves together the scarlet threads of my story, your story...HER story. An ancient tale of Motherhood to be cherished, celebrated and perpetuated through the annals of time.

PART I- SACRED WOMEN'S BUSINESS
HONORING THE DIVINE FEMININE AND RECLAIMING BIRTH AS SACRED

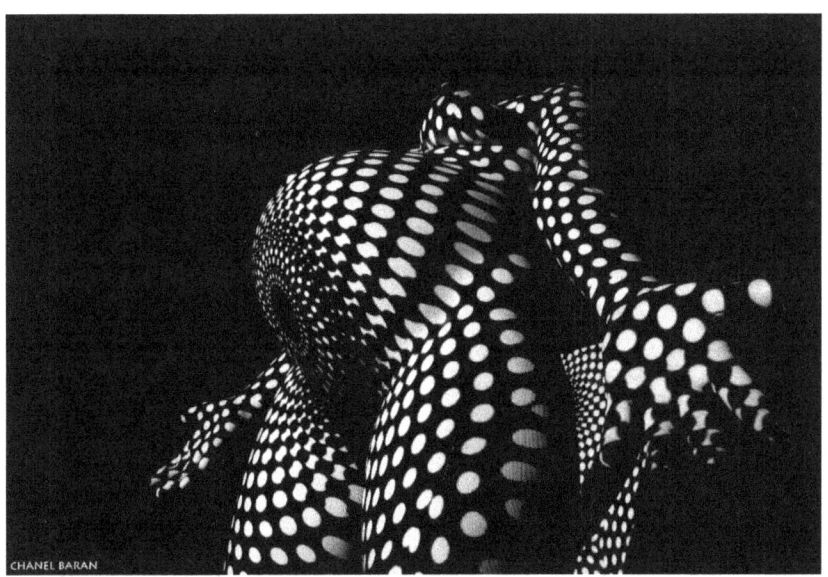

"When enough women realize that birth is a time of great opportunity to get in touch with their true power, and when they are willing to assume responsibility for this, we will reclaim the power of birth and help move technology where it belongs–in the service of birthing women, not their master." -Christiane Northrup, M.D

1

HERSTORY

ATTUNING TO THE WISDOM OF THE WOMEN'S MYSTERIES

"In the world's oldest creation myths, the female god creates the world out of her own body. The Great Mother everywhere was the active and autonomous creatrix of the world."
-Monica Sjöö

The women's mysteries encompass a rich tapestry of teachings, practices and rituals that honour and celebrate the sacredness of women's experiences in relationship to the divine feminine. These mysteries are passed down from generation to generation, providing empowerment, connection and spiritual growth for women worldwide.

The most important and central aspects of the women's mysteries are the recognition of the seasons of womanhood and the power of the menstrual cycle as a symbol of fertility, creativity and connection to the rhythms of nature, birth, death and rebirth. This collective experience of bleeding women is affectionately called the '*Red Thread*' and is woven throughout '*HER*' story, where the womb and the menstrual cycle become sources of wisdom, power and spiritual connection.

Another important aspect of women's mysteries is the celebration of menarche, childbirth, motherhood and menopause, which are sacred rites of passage. Women are honoured for their role as creators and nurturers of life and recognised as the keepers of life's mysteries. The Women's mysteries emphasise a deep connection between women, their wombs and the natural and magical world. Women are seen as inherently connected to the Earth's rhythms, seasons, cycles and expressions of the Goddess in all her forms.

Through cultivating sisterhood, women come together in circles, gatherings and ceremonies to share wisdom and mythology, support each other, create rituals to honour their rites of passage and celebrate the unique gifts and strengths of being women.

Embracing the Seasons of Woman

In the grand tapestry of life, the seasons of woman and the wheel of the year are threads woven together in the fabric of eternity. Each phase of the journey holds its unique beauty and wisdom, guiding us toward self-discovery and transformation. Just as nature ebbs and flows through growth, fruition, decay and rebirth cycles, so does a woman's journey unfold in stages marked by transitions and transformations.

Imagine a wheel turning ceaselessly, its spokes reaching out to touch the essence of each season, mirroring the phases of a woman's life. From the innocence of spring to the deep wisdom of winter, you can traverse landscapes of experience, navigating the ever-shifting terrain of your being, initiated into each season by your blood, which gives colour to the red thread, weaving all women across all timelines- into the very fabric of womanhood.

Standing at the centre of this wheel, you can return home to yourself fully embodied.

The Four Phase Approach

The traditional Triple Goddess mythology of Maiden, Mother and Crone has historically served as a symbolic framework for understanding the stages of a woman's life. However, with increased life expectancy, diverse life paths, delayed parenthood and multi-faceted identities, this model may not fully capture the complexity of women's experiences in modern times.

The extended life span and diverse roles women pursue challenge the linear progression of Maiden, Mother and Crone, calling for a more inclusive and flexible framework. The concept of the four phases of womanhood offers a more dynamic perspective that acknowledges the diversity of women's experiences and their multiple roles throughout their lives.

The four-phase approach, including the stages of Maiden, Mother, Maga and Crone, is an expanded framework developed to offer a more nuanced understanding of women's life stages. While it's difficult to attribute its development to a single individual, it has emerged through the collective exploration and reimagining of traditional feminine archetypes. This approach has been embraced by contemporary scholars, writers and practitioners seeking to honour women's diverse experiences and roles in modern society.

So, let's explore this four-phase approach.

NB: Please keep in mind the ages listed below are generalised and based upon the average female life expectancy of 85 years, equating to roughly 20 years in each phase- except for Maiden- as it would also have to include childhood. The average age of menstruation is 12 years. Also, note that every woman is different in her hormonal journey and choices in life. For this reason, I felt it necessary to start the Mother season at 25 years old, as it coincides with the maturation of the prefrontal cortex and the brain's frontal lobe.

Maiden: The Blossoming Woman

- **Season:** Spring
- **Age:** 12
- **Rite of Passage:** Menarche (first bleed)
- **Qualities:** sexual innocence, fertility, self-serving, beginning self-discovery, optimistic, creative experimentation, curious, playful, receptive, energetic and impressionable.

- **Shadow:** Naive, promiscuous, reckless, thoughtless, timid, unsure of self, porous boundaries, impatient and gullible.

As the first blush of blood graces her, a young girl embarks on a journey of profound transformation, her body whispering ancient secrets of the red thread through the alchemy of menstruation. In this rite of passage, she begins to feel the rhythmic pulse of life within her, awakening to the power of her own unique essence. Like a delicate shoot breaking through the soil, she rises to greet the spring of her existence as a Maiden. She embodies both the light of innocence and the dawning of wisdom, a living paradox of simplicity and depth.

Playful curiosity in her steps and a thirst for knowledge and experience propel her forward. In the sanctuary of her innocence, she explores the sensuality of her emerging womanhood, each sensation a revelation, each discovery a piece of the puzzle of herself. She is fertile ground for creativity and her mind is a fertile field where ideas sprout and flourish. She delights in the myriad ways she can express her blossoming self as her womb becomes activated.

The Maiden is the dawn of womanhood, her journey a sacred pilgrimage toward self-knowledge and empowerment. She is the morning dew on new leaves, the first light that breaks the darkness. Through her, we witness the miracle of growth and the magic of transformation. She is the promise of spring, the embodiment of life's perpetual renewal and a living testament to the simple and profound beauty of becoming.

Mother: The Creatrix/Wild Daughter

- **Season:** Summer
- **Age:** 25+
- **Rite of Passage:** Pregnancy/Childbirth (physical or purpose work)
- **Qualities:** Sacred bridge, gatekeeper, child rearing, nurturing, organised, receptive, intuitive, serving family, career building, Strong and capable, sensual.

- **Shadow:** Militant, rigid, controlling, degrades/depletes selfhood (put needs of others first)

Summer arrives in a blaze of glory and as the wheel turns in this busy season of life, a woman steps into the archetype of the Mother. She embodies the fullness of her power, ripe with the vitality of creation energy. Like the earth yielding its bounty to the sun, she embraces the roles of caregiver and nurturer with grace and responsibility. Her fertility is not solely tied to her womb but to *the way* she expresses herself in the world, weaving her essence into every act of creation.

She embodies creativity and purpose, nurturing children, her career and her community. Her sensuality is deeply rooted, a testament to her inner fire and life force. She is a living paradox, a wild daughter and creatrix combining the Maiden's innocence with the Mother's wisdom, each breath infused with the rhythm of life, every heartbeat a testament to the enduring legacy of love and devotion.

In this busy season of abundance, the Mother celebrates the budding fruits of her labour, basking in the warmth of family, community and connection. She also learns to advocate for her own needs whilst tending to the needs of others, and will often fell the contraction and expansion of life as she continues the process of becoming the Mother she is meant to be.

Maga: The Loving Matriarch

- **Season**: Autumn
- **Age:** 45+
- **Rite of Passage:** Perimenopause/Menopause
- **Qualities:** Coming home to self after children/career- embodying power and sensuality- serving the community, philanthropy and introspection.
- **Shadow:** Bitterness, frustrated by stifled creativity, vanity, manipulative, lonely (empty nest), needy or bitter.

Within the passage of time, autumn arrives with the whispering of endings and new beginnings. Here, a woman steps into the role of the loving matriarch, her spirit tempered by the fires of transformation and life's experiences. As she transitions through this season of reflection and introspection, she gathers the harvest of her years, savouring the memories and lessons that have shaped her journey.

Like falling leaves surrendering to the Earth, she embraces the cycle of rebirth, knowing that the seeds of renewal come from every ending. She learns to grieve and let go of how life used to be, what no longer serves or is in alignment with her dreams and desires and begins to create space for a new depth to emerge in her. This newfound spaciousness is necessary to shift her focus towards her future phases of life, planning for retirement and, ultimately, death. From the stillness that naturally arises in her, she may begin to question her life's path and feel called to seek and explore opportunities she could not previously explore due to her familial commitments. This is a time of waning fertility with the hormonal dance of peri-menopause and creates the necessary initiation into the seat of her unyielding power. She will begin to centre her dreams, desires and needs above others and will be less tolerant of energy that does not foster well-being and fulfilment.

Crone: The Wise Elder

- **Season:** Winter
- **Age:** 65+
- **Rite of Passage:** Retirement
- **Qualities:** Embodied Wisdom, self-confidence, a time to be respected, focus on legacy, honoured and served as an elder and teacher.
- **Shadow:** anti-social, withholding/withdrawal, lost, needy, empty or lonely.

Winter blankets the world in a mantle of stillness as the wheel turns full circle, inviting a woman to journey inward and embrace the wisdom of her years. Here, she embodies the essence of the wise woman, her spirit illuminated by the soft glow of inner knowing. In this season of surrender and release, she embraces the beauty of simplicity and solitude, finding solace in the quiet whispers of the soul.

Like snowflakes falling gently to the ground, she surrenders to the timeless rhythm of the universe. She begins to slow down, enjoy the richness of her legacy and find fulfilling ways to share her inner wisdom and creativity as an elder. Retiring from the flux of life, she becomes a necessary leader that shows younger women the way. In this season, she has more energetic capacity to help and enjoy the wild beauty of children and can playfully share her stories in a way that inspires the next generation to live with wonder and kindness.

It is important for women in this season to make sure they have roots in place to navigate the experiences of an aging body in a way that fosters connection, rather than isolating for fear of becoming burdensome. Crones are our wisdom keepers, our grandmothers who have completed their hormonal journey and become the way-showers through the Women's Mysteries This is also a time for majick as women receive the gifts of their legacy through the expressions of their children, their art and life's work.

Womb Wisdom

The womb is a creative power centre, a place of birth, death and rebirth. Inherently connected to the cyclic nature of the feminine, it is a fertile space to plant the seeds of hope, new life, projects and desires whilst also shedding and releasing those that do not serve us. The womb is a sacred space of deep alchemical majick.

Within the sanctity of our womb, we encounter the whispers of our ancestral lineage, the calling of our innermost desires and the depths of our primal fears. By attuning to the womb's subtle rhythms and energies, we unlock our intuition, creativity, insight and an ancient reservoir of feminine wisdom that guides us through life's process of *becoming*.

For those treading the path towards motherhood, embracing the womb's wisdom becomes necessary for the transition of Maiden into Mother. In the sacred sanctuary of the womb space, women reclaim their sovereignty, ancestral power and inherent creative and sensual expressions. A woman intimately connected to her womb, firmly rooted in the sacred wisdom of her body and soul, will birth with unparalleled presence and power.

Connect With Your Womb

Find a quiet, comfortable space where you won't be disturbed. This could be a cozy corner of your home or a quiet, natural outdoor spot. Sit or lie comfortably, closing your eyes if it feels safe. Take a few deep breaths to relax your body and your jaw and begin to calm your mind.

Gently place your hands on your lower abdomen, over your womb space. Take a moment to connect with the warmth and energy of your hands as they rest over your womb. Bring your awareness to your breath, noticing the rise and fall of your belly with each inhale and exhale. Allow your breath to become slow, deep and rhythmic. Now visualise a warm, golden light radiating from your hands into your womb as you breathe deeply. Imagine this light filling your womb with love, healing and vitality.

Begin to whisper, "I'm here now" and allow yourself to build a relationship with *'her'*... your womb. Take your time to cultivate this presence with your inner realm, tuning in to any sensations, feelings or messages that arise. You may feel a wave of emotion if this is your first time, this is normal. So many women have been living most of their lives disconnected from their body, especially their womb. This simple practice helps you to slowly come home to yourself and the safety and creative power that resides inside your body. Depending on your life's journey and understanding of somatic practice, womb work may be the first revolutionary step towards trusting your intuition and allowing yourself to receive your inner wisdom.

Before concluding your practice, take a moment to express gratitude to your womb for its wisdom, strength and resilience, the connection you've cultivated and the insights you've received.

When you're ready, gently release your hands from your wombspace and take a few more deep breaths to ground yourself. Slowly open your eyes and return your awareness to the present moment, carrying the connection and wisdom of your womb with you.

If you feel called to go deeper in connecting with your womb wisdom and would like to experience a guided journey, you can download my free *Womb Activation Journey* via the link listed in the footnotes below.*

Archetypes

An archetype is a fundamental, universal symbol or pattern that resides in the collective unconscious of humanity. These archetypes manifest in myths, dreams and cultural narratives, representing profound truths and experiences shared across time and space. When we explore these primordial symbols, we touch upon the deepest aspects of the human psyche, connecting with timeless themes and energies that shape our language, perception and understanding of the world and ourselves.

The Oxford Dictionary states that in Jungian Psychology, *'archetype'* means:

> *"A primitive mental image inherited from the earliest human ancestors, and supposed to be present in the collective unconscious."*

So, if these imprints are stored in the collective unconscious, we can access them *at will* when necessary. We can use archetypes as a resource to inspire our creative expressions and serve our best intentions and well-being. The embodiment of feminine archetypes, from ancient to contemporary mythos, changes in expression depending on the behavioural patterns they are expressed through, the cultural narratives they stem from and the language in which they are given form.

Language shapes reality and provides meaning and context to how we perceive and interact with the world. Exploring archetypal energies and expressions becomes a powerful way to connect with different facets of yourself that you may not have permitted yourself to express or even felt were possible to embody. The basic accepted forms of archetypal feminine energies that we've explored so far relate to the neopagan *Triple Goddess* perspective of ancient cultures, comprising the *Maiden, Mother* and *Crone*. Over time, this evolved to the four-phase approach to include

---

* www.donnaraymond.com.au/wombactivationjourney.

the archetype of Maga, which speaks to the experiences of modern women.

As an educator, I've delved into various archetypes (there are many) and realised that fully defining these energies for others can hinder their true expression. Providing rigid definitions distorts the purity of these divine expressions and limits individuals who seek to explore and express these energies freely and creatively through Gnosis. It's important to allow space to engage with these archetypes in your own way, tapping into the energetic signature of their expressions and embracing the natural flow of energy as it emerges through you in the moment. Many archetypes weave together in symbiosis, fluid and ever-changing... Such is the nature of the feminine.

The Eternal Maternal: Archetypal Expressions of the Goddess

Throughout history, goddesses have embodied many qualities, reflecting unique facets of womanhood and maternal energy. Delving into mythological stories and goddess archetypes, we uncover fertility themes, life and death cycles and the importance of nurturing the hearth and home. These narratives offer profound insights into the roles and responsibilities of mothers as nurturers, caretakers and guardians of life.

Diverse representations of the divine feminine provide a rich tapestry of wisdom for women embracing motherhood. Learning from goddess mythology is valuable because these archetypal expressions can inspire us in many ways. They give us strength, wisdom and power, providing timeless examples of navigating life's challenges with grace and resilience. The ever-changing nature of the feminine is beautifully illustrated in these myths, reminding us of the dynamic and multifaceted aspects of womanhood. Before we walk forward we must honour those who walked before us, and the stories held close to their hearts and passed on down the line.

The Primordial Mother

In the vast tapestry of mythology, few themes resonate as deeply and universally as motherhood. From the dawn of human storytelling, mothers have been revered as sources of life, nurturers, protectors and sometimes even figures of destruction, awe and fear. Their stories echo through the ages, weaving together themes of love, sacrifice, strength and wisdom.

In many ancient mythologies, the concept of the primordial mother figure emerges, often depicted as a creator goddess or a symbol of fertility and abundance. This archetype represents the foundational force from which all life springs forth, embodying the creative power of the cosmos. She is the earth's mother, the giver of sustenance and vitality, nurturing all living beings with her boundless love and generosity. The primordial mother symbolises divine femininity, embodying the cycles of birth, growth, death and rebirth. She reminds us of the interconnectedness of all living things and the sacredness of life itself. Through her mythic presence, we find inspiration and guidance in embracing our capacity for creation, nurturing and renewal.

Ancient Mother Goddesses

- **Inanna:** known as Ishtar in later Akkadian and Babylonian mythology, is a revered goddess associated with love, fertility and war. As the queen of the heavens, Inanna embodies the dual nature of femininity, representing both motherhood's nurturing aspect and the warrior's fierce power. Inanna's mythology includes tales of her descent into the underworld, symbolising the cyclical nature of life, death and rebirth. As a fertility goddess, Inanna is often invoked by women seeking blessings for pregnancy, childbirth and nurturing their families. Her presence in ancient Sumerian rituals and hymns underscores her enduring significance as a feminine power and fertility symbol.
- **Hathor:** An ancient Egyptian goddess associated with love, music, dance and fertility. Revered as the 'Mistress of Life,' Hathor embodies the nurturing and life-giving qualities of the divine feminine. She is often depicted as a cow goddess or a woman with cow horns, symbolising her association with fertility and abundance. Hathor is believed to protect women

during childbirth and ensure the well-being of mothers and their children. Her presence in Egyptian religious rituals and ceremonies underscores her role as a benevolent and nurturing mother figure, guiding her devotees through the cycles of life and fertility.

- **Demeter:** The Greek goddess of agriculture, fertility and the harvest. She is best known for her role as the mother of Persephone, who was abducted by Hades and taken to the underworld, leading to Demeter's grief and the seasonal cycle of winter. Demeter is often depicted as a nurturing and protective mother figure, representing the fertility of the earth and the cycle of life, death and rebirth.
- **Isis:** One of the most revered goddesses in ancient Egyptian mythology, associated with motherhood, magic and wisdom. She is the wife of Osiris and the mother of Horus, embodying the ideal of motherhood and family. Isis is often depicted nursing her son Horus, symbolising her role as a nurturing and protective mother figure who guides her child through life's challenges.
- **Yemanja:** A prominent deity in the Yoruba religion and also known as Yemaya. She is the goddess of the sea, motherhood and fertility, often depicted as a nurturing and compassionate figure. Yemanja is believed to be the mother of all Orishas (deities) and is revered for her protective and nurturing qualities, particularly toward her children and devotees.
- **Frigg:** The Norse goddess of marriage, fertility and motherhood. She is also the queen of the Aesir gods, the wife of Odin and the mother of Baldr. Frigg embodies the ideal of a protective and nurturing mother. She is often depicted as a wise and compassionate figure, revered for her foresight and knowledge of destiny.
- **Tara:** A Hindu goddess associated with fertility, childbirth and maternal protection. She is often depicted as a compassionate and nurturing mother who aids women during pregnancy and childbirth. Tara is also revered as a

goddess of wisdom and guidance, offering support and protection to her devotees in times of need.
- **Kuan Yin/Guanyin:** A bodhisattva and goddess of compassion in Chinese and East Asian Buddhism. She is often depicted as a motherly figure, embodying the virtues of kindness, mercy and maternal love. Kuan Yin is revered for aiding those in distress, particularly women and children and is considered a protector of mothers and children.
- **Coatlicue:** An Aztec goddess associated with fertility, motherhood and Earth. She is depicted as a fearsome figure with a skirt of serpents and a necklace made of human hearts and hands. Coatlicue represents the duality of creation and destruction, embodying the cycles of life and death and is revered as the mother of the gods, including Huitzilopochtli, the god of war and the sun.
- **Anahita:** An ancient Persian goddess associated with fertility, water and maternal love. She is often depicted as a radiant figure holding a bundle of plants, symbolising fertility and abundance. Anahita is revered as a protector of women and children and a guardian of the waters, essential for life and fertility in agricultural societies.
- **Mawu-Lisa:** A creator deity in West African mythology, particularly among the Fon people of Benin and the Ewe people of Togo. Mawu is the goddess of the moon, fertility and motherhood, while Lisa is the god of the sun and the sky. Mawu-Lisa is often depicted as a nurturing mother who brings fertility to the earth and sustains all living beings, embodying the cyclical nature of life and the cosmos.
- **Freya:** A Norse goddess associated with love, fertility and beauty. She is often depicted as a powerful and independent figure overseeing love and childbirth matters. Freya's connection to fertility is reflected in her association with the earth's abundance and her role in facilitating the cycles of life and growth. She is revered as a protector of women and a guide for those seeking blessings for childbirth and family life.

- **Brigid:** A Celtic goddess associated with healing, fertility and childbirth. Revered as a guardian of hearth and home, Brigid embodies the nurturing and protective qualities of the divine feminine. She is often invoked by women seeking blessings for fertility, pregnancy and childbirth, as well as protection during the vulnerable stages of motherhood.

Triple Goddess Mythology

A concept deeply ingrained in ancient mythologies and folklore, representing the three distinct phases of the female life cycle: *Maiden, Mother* and *Crone*. Each phase symbolises unique qualities and experiences, with Maidens embodying youth and independence, Mothers representing fertility and nurturing, and Crones embodying wisdom and introspection.

Across different cultures and mythological traditions, the Triple Goddess is depicted in various forms. For instance, in Celtic mythology, the Irish goddess Brigid embodies the three phases of inspiration and creativity, fertility and nurturing, and wisdom and prophecy. In Greek mythology, the goddess Hecate is associated with the moon and magic, childbirth and protection, death and transformation. In Wiccan and Neopagan traditions, the Triple Goddess is often represented by the three lunar phases: the waxing crescent (Maiden), the full moon (Mother), and the waning crescent (Crone). This symbolism reflects life's cyclical nature and the feminine divine's interconnectedness with the cycles of the moon and the natural world.

Harnessing the Power Within

As women, we are the keepers of the mysteries, the carriers of the sacred red thread and the internal flame that ignites the path of transformation. Within the depths of our wombs lies the wisdom of generations, the power of creation and the magic of life itself. Here, in the sacred space of our bodies, we connect with the primal forces of the universe, with the goddesses who have walked before us and with the archetypes that shape our journey.

But beyond the myths and archetypes lies a deeper truth. A truth that speaks to the essence of who we are as women. It is a truth calling upon us to reclaim our power, honour our bodies and embrace the wisdom within. It is a truth that invites us to step into our fullness, to trust in the mystery of life and to surrender to the flow of creation.

As we journey deeper into the mysteries of womanhood, we remember that we are not alone. We walk this path together, hand in hand with our sisters, our mothers and our ancestors. And as we reclaim our divine feminine wisdom, we pave the way for future generations. We must embrace the sacred journey that lies before us, honouring the wisdom of our bodies, the magic of our wombs and the power of our birthing.

TOGETHER, we step boldly into the light of our divine feminine essence, knowing that we are strong, wise, and infinitely capable of creating our desired world. To shine our light bright, we must not turn away from the injustice of the past but rather lean into the shadows and liberate women from the hands of suffering. As hard as that is, as wisdom keepers and cycle breakers, it is necessary to reclaim the future generations' path, to love and bring it back into the hands, hearts and wombs of the women who birth them.

2

ROTTEN ROOTS
THE PARASITIC NATURE OF PATRIARCHAL BIRTH

"Humanizing birth means understanding that the woman giving birth is a human being, not a machine and not just a container for making babies. Showing women- half of all people- that they are inferior and inadequate by taking away their power to give birth is a tragedy for all society."
- Marsden Wagner

A strangler fig, whose seed is dropped into the branches and bark of a host tree, slowly cascades air roots down into the fertile soil below, silently wrapping around and gripping onto the host tree. It eventually suffocates and consumes the host, until it dies. They do this in dark forests as a way to compete for light.

If you didn't know any better, if you didn't have the eyes to see the truth, you would perceive the fig as robust and resilient, all the while completely unaware of the host tree, that over time, became invisible, enveloped in darkness and forgotten because it was forced to bear the weight of this parasite's thirst for light.

Just like the parasitic fig, such is the nature of Patriarchal birth. To go deep into understanding how our culture has adopted this perspective that birth is unsafe, painful and risky and how women have been slowly brainwashed into not trusting their innate body wisdom and the natural beauty of birth is one of the most profound initiations a woman will ever embark upon. We have to trace these stories back to their roots... as rotten as they are. When we know better, we do better.

When we lean in and take a closer look at the suffering our foremothers endured, we can grieve this pain and loss and liberate our lineage from this suffering by awaken the power of our womb and choose a new way of birthing with phenomenal power.

Reject the System

The current birthing environment is one steeped in fear, mistreatment and disconnection. The birthing field has been infiltrated by a desire to penetrate and control *The Great Mystery* of birth. The Women's Mysteries.

What we see today is the breeding of a parasitic system of unnecessary intervention, lack of informed consent and continuity of care, whereby women are handing over their power because they have been taught to not trust their body's ability to give birth, which in the majority of cases is and should be a natural and safe physiological process.

I'm not advocating that the medical establishment be completely rejected. Of course, it has its place when necessary and for some women and their babies, it is necessary and can be life-saving. From my perspective, what I witness is a Machiavellian machine coercing new parents into a system of oppression, which often leaves families traumatised by what should be a blissful and joyous expression of union and love. To manipulate, disempower and control birth by taking it out of the hands of women and placing it into the constructs of fear is the ultimate act of terrorism, misogyny and violence against humanity.

CURRENT STATISTICS SHOW that in Australia, 1 in 10 women are reported to experience PTSD after a traumatic birth, and 1 in 3 women experience birth intervention. Birth trauma not only affects the mental health of the mother and imprints on the baby and family members, but it also affects our maternal care providers... our midwives and doulas.

According to a survey conducted by The Members of the Australian College of Midwives, More than two-thirds of midwives (67.2%) reported having witnessed a traumatic birth event that included interpersonal care-related trauma features. Midwives recalled strong emotions during or shortly after witnessing the traumatic birth event, such as feelings of horror (74.8%) and guilt (65.3%) about what happened to the woman. Midwives who witnessed birth trauma that included care-related features were significantly more likely to recall peritraumatic distress, including feelings of horror and guilt, than midwives who witnessed non-interpersonal birth trauma. 17% of midwives met the criteria for probable posttraumatic stress disorder. Witnessing abusive care was associated with more severe posttraumatic stress than other types of trauma. [1]

Looking at those statistics from the perspective of birth workers, you can see the bigger picture of what birthing mothers and families are experiencing before, during and after birth. Unfortunately, the unnecessary over-medicalisation of birth within the 'system' has led to a disconnect from the holistic nature of birth being an initiatory journey that is deeply intimate and sacred.

When the focus is isolated to the physical 'outcome' of pregnancy resulting in a live baby and mother, the very foundation of birth being a sacred experience is desecrated because the whole journey is deeply emotional, psychological and spiritual for the mother and baby. We're talking about the foundational imprints of a soul's entry into this world and the connection a mother has to creation energy and her power as a bridge between worlds. Birth Matters.

Unfortunately, our current system does not foster a woman's spiritual relationship with her baby and power as a mother. So much fear and misinformation surrounds such a natural and normal physiological process. The biggest fear is that something will go wrong and lead to complications or the death of either a baby, a new mother or worse, both. Yes, maternal death is a fact; it can happen, but did you know that one of the leading causes of maternal death in Australia is suicide?

Can you take a moment to sit with that and what that means? It means that the current system is failing women. It means the damaging effects of birth traumas are real. It means that women are suffering in silence. This is Spiritual warfare!

The easiest way to create and breed passive consumers and slaves to the system is by corrupting the blueprint of conscious birthing, the primal codes for safe, peaceful and equanimous birth that hold the fabric of the sacred bond between mother and child. Control the birth, control the culture.

It wasn't always this way though. Birth was considered sacred women's business, attended by midwives and community-wise women as men were not allowed access to the mysteries of childbirth. The word midwife is derived from the Old English word *mid*, 'with' and *wif*, 'woman', and translates to '*with-woman.*'

Women supported women in giving birth at home. The birth was seen as a natural rite of passage for women, and the codes remained intact as they had been for thousands of years.

So, what was the turning point?

How did we go from women giving birth on country and at home, supported by women, to the over-medicalised hospital birth practices we have now? Let's take a look back towards those who have walked before us.

Risky Business

In her research paper titled, *The Evolution of Maternal Birthing Position,*[2] published in the American Journal of Public Health, Lauren Dundes, MHS, explores the relationship between horizontal birthing positions and the rise of physician and obstetric-led births.

What can be deduced from this research is that there was indeed an agenda to infiltrate the birthing space, which was traditionally reserved for women-centric practice and attended only by midwives.

All over the world, women have adopted more upright birthing positions such as squatting, kneeling, sitting and standing, using the natural pull of gravity to birth their babies. During the early to late 1500s, controversial birthing positions such as the dorsal and lithotomy positions were adopted, which placed birthing women on their backs and a side laying position was commonly adopted by many women, except those in rural settings.

Perhaps the most influential figure in changing the attitudes towards birth and thus favouring a more medicalised approach to labour was 16th-century physician Francois Mauriceau, who advocated for reclined birthing as it was supposedly more comfortable for women and gave better access to the physician attending the birth.

It is interesting to note that in Dundes's article, she mentions that Mariceau perceived the process of childbirth as an illness, claiming that pregnancy was a "tumour of the belly" and, through his beliefs, perpetuated the narrative that defined birth as pathological and abnormal.

IF BIRTH WERE CONSIDERED a natural and physiological process, as many village midwives knew, physicians, surgeons and the new profession of obstetricians would be out of business. Women knew back then as much as they do now, that horizontal birthing is an unnatural position that can lead to more discomfort, pain and an increased risk of intervention. How convenient it was for a rising profession of men who were largely only permitted access into the birthing space if there was a need for a medical emergency due to a high risk of an infant or maternal mortality because, at the time, men in the women's birthing space were considered indecent.

The popularity of horizontal birthing gained momentum, presumably from King Louis XIV, who was said to have had a fixation on wanting to view his heirs being born as was previously unable to witness this from the traditional birthing stools used in France. Following the influence of Mariceau, the expectant mother was laid flat on her back with legs and hips spread open and wide, giving the King the full, unrestricted viewing pleasure of having his child born. It is also said that he invited others into the room to watch. This was a standard practice for royals throughout Europe at the time.

Stories have been passed down that this type of birth (as you can imagine) was incredibly painful for the mother, which not only increased complications due to the unnatural position, it also increased the need for medical intervention, often with the baby being forcibly removed, thus birth was deemed too risky to be left in the hands of women.

The battle for business began and the art of Midwifery and natural birth was usurped by the science of Obstetrics. Women no longer birthed babies, men delivered them. Fear tainted the collective consciousness of women and this new perspective of birth being a painful disorder that women must endure, inoculated the consciousness of women throughout Europe to the point that many women would seek ways to escape the immense pain that was now associated with giving birth, as if this was now our birthright.

Anarcha

In Alabama, in 1845, a young enslaved girl named Anarcha, aged between thirteen and seventeen years old, went into labour. Due to unknown complications, after three days, plantation physician James Marion Sims arrived to assist the young woman he called *'little mulatto girl'*[3],* by using iron forceps to pull her baby out. A procedure he had no previous experience with. Sims went on to continue this practice on other enslaved women, which resulted in infant fatalities.

After the stillbirth, Anarcha was sent to see Sims again to help with her vesicovaginal fistula, unhealed tears in her vagina and rectum. This caused her to suffer from excruciating pain as she had uncontrollable incontinence and bowel movements, which would seep into her open wounds, leading to infection, inflammation and a foul odour. You can imagine how embarrassing and isolating this would be to deal with on its own, not including the grief from losing a child and the trauma from a painfully long labour with intervention- one which likely caused her injury.

Sims requested Anarcha to kneel on all fours on his examination table and proceeded to perform his first experimental surgical attempt to cure the fistula without anaesthesia or any explanation of what he was doing. This would be the start of many experimental, nonconsensual

---

* **Mulatto (noun)** usually offensive: the first-generation offspring of a black person and a white person

operations on enslaved women at the hands of Sims. It is known that Sims operated on at least twelve unnamed women; of those, two were later known as Betsy and Lucy. It is documented that Sims did allow the women opium during their recovery but only provided them with minimal food.

James Marion Sims performed over thirty experimental, nonconsensual operations without anesthesia on Anarcha before successfully closing the fistula and tears. He later became famous for his work and travelled all over the country, treating white women who were considered unable to tolerate the pain of surgery and so administered ether for pain relief. He is celebrated as the 'Father of Modern Gynaecology'.

Disconnected: Anesthesia and Twilight Sleep

After years of requesting access to pain relief for childbirth, finally, in 1853, Queen Victoria was administered chloroform by her physician, Dr John Snow. Up until this point in time, anesthesia was reserved only for surgical procedures and as a relatively new practice, it was quite taboo to use in childbirth. However, after the royal birth, it ended any moral objection to the practice and represented a new sense of freedom for women to experience a pain-free birth.

Fast forward to early 1902 in Freiburg, Germany, a new promise of pain-free childbirth hit the market. Originally suggested as a form of surgical anaesthesia, branching off from his peers, Carl Gauss began to slowly develop the *'Dämmerschlaf'*, also known as the *Freiburg method*, aka *Twilight Sleep*.

Twilight Sleep was a method of administering psychoactive drugs to induce a state of pain relief whilst creating amnesia so the birthing mother would not remember the pain of childbirth. A powerful mixture of morphine and scopolamine was injected frequently, providing a potent cocktail of chemicals, leaving women semi-conscious during labour, often with no recollection of the birth at all, which of course disrupts the mother's natural maternal instinct and bonding with her baby.

The amount of morphine used was meant to create pain relief, though it often resulted in women losing their inhibitions during labour and the scopolamine would often result in psychotic episodes. Due to the effects of the narcotics, women were often restricted, strapped to beds by their wrists and ankles to prevent them from injuring themselves or birth attendants. They were left in 'labour cribs' bound and screaming for as long as it took for labour to come to completion.

A New York Times article published in 1915 promoted the method to a wider audience, stating, *"Through twilight sleep, a new era has dawned for woman and through her for the whole human race."*[4] With no memory afterwards, the method delivered the promise to mothers of 'pain-free' childbirth.

As you can imagine, the drugs also affected the newborn baby as they would cross the placental barrier and enter the central nervous system. Consequentially, babies were born drugged with respiratory issues and often needed medical assistance to be revived. It is said that this is the reason babies were held upside down and spanked upon arrival in the outside world. The practice was widely used and accepted until the mid-1960s when a new wave of natural, un-medicated childbirth practices was preferred.

Barbaric Birth Practices

Chainsaw

Did you know that the chainsaw was first invented in 1780 by two Scottish doctors, John Aitken and James Jeffray and was used to cut through women's pelvises to deliver babies without anaesthetic? A hand-cranked chainsaw with fine-cutting teeth was used to cut through cartilage and ligaments to extract a baby that was considered too big or obstructed-keep in mind many of these women were on their backs during labour. In the late 19th century, the chainsaw was mechanised to increase ease of use upon expectant mothers and was then superseded by the Gigli saw, which was also used for amputating limbs, along with decaying flesh and bones, both of which are still used in some parts of the world where cesarean is unavailable.

Symphysiotomy

Symphysiotomy is an outdated, dangerous surgical procedure in which the cartilage of the pubic symphysis is unhinged and divided to widen the pelvis by approximately 2cm to help with obstructed labour. It is also known as a pelviotomy and synchondrotomy.

First advocated in 1597 by Severin Pineau, it became a routine surgical procedure that carried risks of urethral and bladder injury, fistulas, infection, pain and long-term difficulty walking. Ireland was the only country in the Western world to practise these mutilating operations in modern times and it is estimated that 1,500 women unknowingly and without consent underwent symphysiotomies during childbirth between 1944 and 1987. Irish politician Gerry Adams described the procedure as, "Institutional abuse involving acts of butchery against women."

In 2012, in front of the Joint Oireachtas Committee on Justice, Margaret Conlan, who was operated upon in 1962 in St Finbarr's Hospital, Cork, testified that she had never been told anything about it: "My baby's head was perforated, and the baby died... I did not find out [about the symphysiotomy] until I read it in the newspaper."[5]

Husband Stitch

The concept of the Husband Stitch is to add an extra stitch whilst suturing a woman's perineum following an episiotomy or tear to make the vagina 'tighter' and increase pleasure for a male partner during penetrative sex. This can often lead to ongoing pain and discomfort, especially during intercourse.

Although there are no studies to show how many women have been affected by this procedure, there are countless stories from women around the world where this procedure was done without knowledge or permission, often said to be accompanied by unprofessional comments or jokes by medical practitioners. This is considered medical abuse, though women have difficulty proving it.

> "The fact that there is even a practice called the husband stitch is a perfect example of the intersection of the objectification of women's

bodies and healthcare. As much as we try to remove the sexualization of women from appropriate obstetric care, of course, the patriarchy is going to find its way in there."

— STEPHANIE TILLMAN- CERTIFIED NURSE MIDWIFE

History of Reproductive Rights

Medieval hospitals were very different to what we know today. They were charitable institutions designed to care for the sick, poor, needy and women in unstable domestic situations. Most women birthed at home with a midwife because the hospitals were to take care of sick people and the consensus was that birth was not an illness, so it was dealt with at home, thus reducing the risk of passing on disease and infection. Poor unmarried women, however, often ended up in the hospitals with nowhere else to go and due to their social situation, often meant that their babies were left abandoned and taken care of by wet nurses.

Throughout the Middle Ages, midwives were expected to be moral judges, looking out for instances of illegitimate births and infanticide, which was often practised during times of famine. They were more experienced in the birthing spaces compared to their male counterparts, though they were paid poorly, with the added threat of being suspected of witchcraft for herbal concoctions to aid or terminate a pregnancy and the use of rituals and relics for protection.

Contraception choices varied from ancient to medieval times, with the use of abortifacient herbs and spermicides, condoms (external and internal) made of animal bladders and intestines, concoctions of heavy metals like mercury, lead and arsenic, barrier methods using sponges and moss and vaginal douching. The most common method was *coitus interruptus*- the withdrawal/pull-out method, which has an efficacy rate of approximately 75%. In medieval Western Europe, however, any attempt to cease or prevent pregnancy was deemed immoral by the Catholic Church.

In 1918 Vienna, many women's health suffered considerably during and after the First World War as men were conscripted and women were left to pick up the slack to provide for the family unit on their own, often waiting in line for hours to receive food rations. Although the birth rate declined across many countries due to the war and economic hardship, those who did become pregnant were often too weak to carry or birth a child safely and a rise in miscarriages and infant mortality affected women in many areas.

Abortions were illegal in Austria and Germany at the time, although women considered this a valid method of preventing an already difficult situation from getting worse. In those days, common abortifacient herbs like pennyroyal, savin juniper and ergot were used, as well as chemicals and other instruments, which often led to injury and infection, making abortion a life-threatening process. This was a risk some women were willing to take, even with the looming fear of five years imprisonment if caught.

When we look back to the past to acknowledge where we have come from, what life was like for women in the last few centuries and what emotions children have been imprinted with, we can start to see a larger and more sinister pattern of disconnect and disempowerment.

SOME QUESTIONS TO PONDER:

- How many babies have been imprinted with violence and fear, consequently disconnected from the gentle ways of birth and bonding with the Mother?
- How many generations of families have felt unsafe after being displaced through slavery, war and socio-political agendas?
- How many women were forced or coerced into pregnancy, even when facing the risks of injury, infection or death?
- How did these pregnancies and births affect the generations of children born during these times?
- How does this relate to the way that we, as a collective, treat the Earth?

Can you see the bigger picture... a pattern? If your early imprints are of violence and abuse, that is what will be comfortable and familiar to you. Birth is crucial because it sets the foundations of one's definition of love, empathy and comfort. We will explore this in the next chapter.

A Call to Remember

As the veil of a collective amnesia spell gradually lifts, women are awakening to the potency of the women's mysteries and the power of their wombs. Together, we are coming to understand the far-reaching influence of systems engineered to suppress women's wisdom—a suppression fueled by historical, social, and cultural factors deeply rooted in misogyny, disconnection and dominance.

In patriarchal societies, women's roles and knowledge were systematically devalued, relegating them to subordinate positions with limited access to education and leadership, eroding women's spiritual practices, while the medicalisation of childbirth marginalised women's autonomy and intuition in favour of 'safe' medical interventions. This systemic oppression reinforced patriarchal control over women's bodies and experiences, perpetuating the erasure of women's wisdom.

I invite you to take a moment to reflect upon how far we've come and how far we have to go as a collective to liberate women from this unnecessary suffering.

Reclaiming this wisdom is paramount for restoring balance, healing intergenerational trauma and empowering women to reclaim agency over their bodies and births. To achieve this, we must delve into the shadows of the past and acknowledge the trials our foremothers endured. By healing the timelines of HERstory, we can remember our inherent power as wisdom keepers, weave the red thread of revolution and restore the ancient wisdom of the womb to all womankind.

Birthing the New Paradigm

Once you fully comprehend the scope of where we've come from and the trajectory of where we are going, you can make conscious choices about the world you want to invest your time and energy into creating. You need to know the games at play and be able to see the system's subtle programming, you must shine your light into the dark to illuminate the shadows and retain your sovereignty.

More importantly, you must learn to let go of the old stories, tap into your intuition, listen deeply and trust your innate body wisdom as a birthing mother, allowing yourself to draw upon the strength and courage of all birthing mothers who walked before you. Only then will you consciously and purposefully birth without fear.

We can learn from past mistakes to heal HERstory, the stories encoded in our blood and bones, carried by the ancient red thread to ensure we clear the way for future generations. This is our birthright, and it must be fiercely guarded and protected. We are the birthkeepers of the new dawn.

As THE LATE author and midwife *Jeannine Parvati Baker said,*
"Peace on Earth begins with Birth."

3

RIPPLES OF LOVE
THE IMPACT OF BIRTH EXPERIENCES

*"To change the world, we must first change
the way the babies are being born."*
-Michel Odent

The journey from conceiving to birthing a child and onwards into motherhood, in my opinion, is *the* most important work in the world. It's not because you are growing organs and limbs within your body; that's pretty important and phenomenal. It's because Mothers are responsible for imprinting the consciousness of a new child.

As a parent and primary caregiver, you are responsible for shaping and programming the consciousness and reality of your child.

I don't believe this journey is a mere accident for one second. If this is the first time you've tuned into that perspective, then I encourage you to sit with what it means on a much larger scale and then you will understand the scope of this great work and your role in it.

THIS IS A BIG DEAL, being a Mother is a big deal... You are a big deal!

The Great Work

Every thought, emotion and action an expectant mother expresses is transmitted to her child in utero. At the moment of birth, a baby imprints everything it needs to know about life and love via sensory information provided by the Mother. However, the birth experience itself can introduce complexities, particularly in settings that diverge from the natural rhythms of undisturbed childbirth. The stark transition from the womb's warmth and security to the world's harshness can imprint feelings of uncertainty and distress, shaping the child's perception of love from the outset and as such, harsh realities need to be met with honesty and compassion because when we know better, we make better choices. When we know better, we work with what we've got and do our best within the frameworks we operate. That is why education is the key to empowerment.

To put this harshness into perspective, imagine for a moment you are a newborn baby in the stereotypical Western model of a clinical and medicalised birth setting, assuming for a moment it's a drug-free, head-down vaginal birth.

As labour begins you begin to feel as though you are leaving the safety of your home, the warm and dark womb, with its muffled sounds and constant nurturing and nutrients. Suddenly, things begin to constrict around you, the space becomes tighter and there is this immense pressure around your little body- particularly your skull, as your bones shift and mould. Is this what death feels like? You begin to feel the constriction squeezing you as you move through the birth canal, slowly emerging into a completely foreign and cold environment, bright lights, smells and loud noises and then all of a sudden you are whisked away from everything you've ever known, Mother.

Your line of nutrition is severed almost immediately. You are weighed, measured, quickly and aggressively wiped down, wrapped up and then handed to your bewildered mother; both of you are completely disorientated at this pivotal moment of your arrival. Welcome to the world, little one; you're in for one hell of a ride!

In his book, *A Birth Without Violence,* French obstetrician and author Fredrerik Leboyer describes this process with empathic detail. Understanding birth from the child's perspective and the emotional impact of this critical moment will help us all make better choices, even within the Western model of medicalised birth practices. This is paramount to leaving a legacy of trust, connection, empathy and love for future generations.

The great work is restoring the codes of peaceful and conscious birth as a sacred initiation to imprint the new generations of mothers and children with love, connection, respect and kindness. Empowered mothers empower their children, who then go on to have empowered births, so on and so forth.

Slowly, we are remembering.

Nurturing Neurology: The Impact of Maternal Experiences on Fetal Nervous System

During pregnancy, the baby's nervous system develops in the early embryonic stages and then progresses throughout gestation. By the end of the second trimester, fundamental brain and spinal cord structures are already established. Throughout pregnancy, different components of the baby's nervous system, such as the brain, sensory systems, motor control and autonomic functions, are active and evolving. These initial neurological processes form the basis for the baby's growth, behaviour and responses following birth. However, this development is significantly influenced by other factors, particularly the mother's experiences during pregnancy.

By the end of the first trimester, basic structures such as the cerebral cortex, which is responsible for higher cognitive functions and the brainstem, which controls basic bodily functions like breathing and heart rate are present. As pregnancy progresses, more complex brain regions develop such as the hippocampus for memory and learning and the amygdala for emotional processing.

By the second trimester, sensory systems begin to function. The auditory system is one of the earliest to become active, with the baby able to hear sounds from the outside world. This includes the mother's voice, heartbeat and other ambient sounds. The visual system also starts to develop, although the eyes remain closed until later in pregnancy. Babies may respond to light and darkness even in utero. Motor Neurons and pathways responsible for movement begin to develop early in pregnancy. By the second trimester, the baby starts to make spontaneous movements, such as kicking and stretching. These movements become more coordinated as the nervous system continues to mature.

The autonomic nervous system, responsible for regulating involuntary bodily functions like heart rate, digestion and breathing, also becomes active in utero. This system helps maintain homeostasis and responds to internal and external stimuli, ensuring the baby's physiological needs are met even before birth.

A mother's emotional state can significantly impact her baby's development. High levels of stress and anxiety in the mother can lead to the release of stress hormones like cortisol, which may affect the developing fetal brain. Chronic stress during pregnancy has been linked to adverse outcomes for the baby, including alterations in brain development and increased risk of emotional and behavioural problems later in life.

Additionally, the mother's physical health and lifestyle choices are crucial in her baby's nervous system development. Adequate nutrition, avoidance of harmful substances like alcohol, tobacco and other drugs and access to prenatal care are essential for promoting healthy brain development in the baby. Supportive prenatal care can help reduce maternal stress and anxiety, creating a more nurturing environment for the baby's development.

Limbic Imprinting

Limbic imprinting is a process centred around the brain's limbic system, involving structures like the amygdala, hippocampus, and hypothalamus. Emotional experiences during critical developmental periods, such as infancy and early childhood, shape neural connections within the limbic system and across the brain. Positive experiences trigger the release of neurotransmitters like dopamine and oxytocin, fostering feelings of pleasure, bonding, and trust.

Conversely, negative experiences can lead to stress responses and the release of cortisol. Hormonal regulation, particularly involving oxytocin and cortisol, influences emotional responses and behaviours. Over time, limbic imprinting leaves lasting effects on emotional development, attachment styles and social interactions, with positive experiences promoting secure attachment and adaptive behaviours, while negative experiences can result in insecure attachment and maladaptive emotional responses.

In 2012, I was introduced to the term *Limbic Imprinting*[1] and the work of Elena Tonetti-Vladimirova[2] by my friend Melissa, who was a local doula and *Birth into Being* practitioner at the time. Over 4 days, Melissa facilitated levels 1 and 2 of this work, and our small group of women were guided through a multi-sensory series of exercises that helped to connect us with our birth story and how it continued to play out in our lives and relationships. We then had the opportunity to recode our birth story, connect with our core wounding, reveal our limbic imprint and role-play our brain in action to release old patterns and live more fully embodied. It was deep and profoundly healing work for me at the time as I was grieving the loss of my father.

In 1982, Elena began to work with the Russian waterbirth pioneer Igor Charkovsky to search for ways to eliminate birth trauma. Over time, she became known as a Spiritual Midwife and developed the modality now known as *Birth into Being*, which has helped thousands of people all over the world heal from birth trauma and recode new pathways to giving and receiving love.

In preparation for this book, I reached out to Elena to include her wisdom on limbic imprinting and to quote her directly. As English is her second language, she revised a passage for me to include in this book.

> "To better understand the term '*Limbic Imprint*,' let's look at the basic structure of our brain. At the tip of the spinal cord, there is a segment called the Reptilian brain, responsible purely for the physiological functions of the body. That's the part of the brain that still remains functional when a person is in a coma, for example, in a 'vegetable' state, - the basic physiology of the body is still going on, women even

keep menstruating and can continue with gestation if they are pregnant.

Then there is the Cortex, responsible for our mental activity and cognitive functions: logic, calculating, planning, ability to be responsible, learn new skills, etc.

And then we have the Limbic system of the brain, which governs our emotions and feelings. Limbic Imprinting happens on a cellular level in that part of the brain which is not directly connected with the cortex (responsible for cognitive memory and decision-making). The limbic brain forms halfway through gestation, way earlier than the cortex. During gestation and birth, the limbic system absorbs and registers all of our sensations and feelings, without delivering it to the cognitive part of the brain, simply because the cognitive function does not exist yet. That memory will remain in the body, on a cellular level, throughout the rest of our life, whether we know it or not.

We come into this world wide-open to receive love. When we do receive it, as our first primal experience, our nervous system is limbically imprinted – 'programmed' with the undeniable rightness of being. Being held in the mother's loving arms, feeding from her breast and seeing the great joy in the father's eyes, provides us with the natural sense of bliss and security; it sets the world as the right place for us to be in.

If our first impressions of being in the body are anything less than loving (painful, frightening, lonely...), then that 'anything' imprints as a valid experience of love. It is immediately coded into our nervous system as a 'comfort zone,' acting as a surrogate for the love and nurturing, regardless of how painful and undesirable it actually was. And in the future, as adults, we will unconsciously, automatically re-create the conditions of neglect that were imprinted at birth and through our early childhood. Research done by the pioneers of prenatal psychology, such as: Dr. Thomas Verny, Dr. David Chamberlain, Dr. William Emerson shows that an overwhelming amount of physical conditions and behavioral disorders are the direct result of traumatic gestational experiences and complications during delivery, including unnecessary mechanical interventions and an overdose of anesthesia.

Also, it turns out, on top of the devastating effect of trauma during the actual birth, what happens after it, like routine impersonal postpartum care, is also extremely devastating for the baby: lack of immediate warm, soft and nurturing contact with the mother, premature cutting of the umbilical cord, rude handling, circumcision, needles, bright lights, startling noises... all this sensory overload becomes instantly wired into the newborn's nervous systems as the new 'comfort zone', against all logic, as logic is not developed yet. So that person will continue to unconsciously recreate/attract the same repeated situations of lack of nurturing experiences, even abuse, and/or become abusive. Even if later on in life, his or hers rational mind/cortex will recognize this pattern as 'abuse', the imprinting had already happened in a different part of the brain, which doesn't have the skill to stop the pattern.

The most effective techniques of neutralizing the birth trauma (loose term, as by 'birth trauma' I mean all negative experiences during gestation, birth and early formative period) are the ones that activate all parts of the brain (reptilian, limbic and cortex) at the same time with the same intensity. That is exactly what introduces the new reference point into the nervous system, creating an alternative route for the brain function. When only the Cortex is involved (like in any talk therapy), or only Reptilian brain (as in yoga or any purely physical modality), or only Limbic (as in art expressions, for example), the whole system remains fragmented.

It is very important to do all of those things, we absolutely need all of them, to talk, to understand what's going on with us, to exercise, to move our bodies, to find our favourite artforms of self-expression. But while all of those activities offer powerful ways of COPING without primal trauma, by themselves, they are rarely able to bring the deep shift in our emotional and behavioral patterns on the subconscious level.

The best route is to find a healing modality that affords the aforementioned experience of activating the mind-body-emotion as a unit. Then healing happens very quickly."

— ELENA TONETTI-VLADIMIROVA NOVEMBER, 2006
(REVISED IN 2022 FOR MAIDEN TO MOTHER)

What Is Love?

The concept of 'love' takes on a unique perspective when considering limbic imprinting and the early wiring of the nervous system. In this context, a baby's perception of love is deeply intertwined with its earliest experiences of safety and security, which can be influenced by maternal experiences during pregnancy.

Limbic Imprinting suggests that a baby's understanding of love is shaped by the emotional experiences imprinted during critical periods of development, particularly in utero and during early infancy. These experiences create a blueprint for how the child perceives and responds to love.

However, the complexity arises when considering that the child's earliest imprints of safety may not always align with traditional notions of love. If the mother experienced stress, anxiety or trauma during pregnancy, the baby's nervous system may have been wired to associate love with feelings of uncertainty or distress. This can lead to a skewed perception of love, where the baby may interpret stressful situations as normal or loving.

In such cases the concept of love becomes nuanced, reflecting positive emotions and the interplay of early experiences and neurobiological wiring. It highlights the importance of understanding how maternal experiences during pregnancy can profoundly influence a baby's perception of love and emotional well-being.

Addressing this concept requires acknowledging the complexity of early imprinting and its implications for emotional development. It emphasises the need for creating safe, nurturing environments and support for mothers and babies, laying the foundation for healthy emotional connections and relationships based on genuine love and security.

Origin Stories

Do you know your story of origin? If it is possible, I would encourage you to seek ways to find out what your Mother and Grandmother's pregnancies were like. What was life like for them at the time of their pregnancy?

When a child is in utero, they are fully merged with the Mother as one, energetically and physically, via the placenta. Everything that the mother experiences is imprinted upon her unborn child through sensory information, which helps to program the child to life outside the womb. Between 16-20 weeks gestation, a female fetus will have around 6 to 7 million egg cells (oocytes) in her ovaries. These eggs will gradually die throughout her lifetime, leaving around 1 to 2 million present during sexual maturity. New research suggests stem cells within the ovaries can create new eggs and replenish the egg stock. However, more research is still being conducted into this theory.

Why is this important to note? Well, it is because *you* were once part of one of those oocytes in your mother's ovaries, as she developed inside your grandmother's womb. There is a reason why the Maiden, Mother and Crone dynamic has been respected in ancient symbology.

With the scientific field of Epigenetics[*,3] exploring ways memory is passed down through cellular DNA, it is important to understand this concept of origin stories as you may experience thoughts, beliefs and feelings that aren't your own. Many women will find their matrilineal storylines intact and exploring these stories can be easy as they have been passed down from women in the family line in many different ways. For others, it may be difficult to explore origins as there is a disconnect or severing of the line from womb to womb. This is not to say that discovering these imprints is impossible, indeed, it may prove to be quite the challenge and as they say, where there is a will, there is a way. Sometimes, that means tapping into the answers that lay hidden inside us.

In his book *Voices of the Womb*, Author Michael Gabriel shares insight into the spiritual dimensions of fetal imprinting, whereby through hypnosis, his patients regressed to times inside the womb, the moment of conception and even pre-conception. Under this hypnotic stage of regression, patients experienced and relived the emotions of the mother and were able to identify how this shaped their personality and behaviours outside of the womb. They were even able to pick up on the

---

[*] "Epigenetics is the study of how your behaviors and environment can cause changes that affect the way your genes work. Unlike genetic changes, epigenetic changes are reversible and do not change your DNA sequence, but they can change how your body reads a DNA sequence."

thoughts and emotions of their father, which were absorbed in the mother's energetic field and passed through the womb. Mind-blowing!

This book is a ground-breaking revelation into transpersonal healing and understanding the power of our origin story and how the stories that surrounded our mother, her mother and those in close relationships are passed through the womb, shaping the behaviours and beliefs of the next generation. I feel that this type of work can be quite revealing and healing for those who have lost their connection to their biological mother and I do believe that it is possible to soothe the pain from this disconnection that nurtures the inherent loss and replaces it with a deeper and more integrated sense of value and belonging.

Connecting with your story of origin will help you to walk clearly and gently on the Earth as a conscious custodian and birth-keeper, feeling a deep and innate sense of purpose and belonging.

Know your Birth Story

Branching off from exploring your *Origin Story* is finding out your birth story. The energy surrounding your birth can shape how you show up in the world and how you give birth. When I first made the connection of my creative expressions to my birth story, I was blown away.

My natural creative state had a stop-start energy to it. I would begin with a surge of inspired energy, a sense of urgency feeling activated and in a rush to create whatever was coming through me, then I would procrastinate and retreat and wonder if what I was creating was a priority. Sometimes, I would struggle to see it through to completion. It was incredibly frustrating until I realised it was directly connected to the way my mother's labour and my birth played out.

My mother went into labour early at around 28 weeks, convinced now that it was due to the spraying of crops in the nearby rural Victorian countryside. As the fourth live child to come through her womb, she knew what was happening and went to the local hospital. Faced with the potential of giving birth to a premature baby, she was administered drugs to stop labour from progressing. Many weeks later, she was then actually induced and I was birthed as a post-term baby at 41+2 weeks. So, it makes sense to look at how your birth story plays out and influences you, too.

Here are some questions to sit with and ponder.

- Do you feel rushed or forced to do things you're not ready for?
- Do you feel like you never have a choice in life?
- Do you feel pressured to perform?
- Do you feel like you do things backwards or that opportunities are taken from you at the last minute?

THINK ABOUT THE ENERGY/THEMES and emotions surrounding different birth types. Premature labour, long labours, short labours, use of drugs, inductions, forceps, vacuum, cesarean, emergency procedures, spontaneous, quick births, breach, nuchal cord, shoulder dystocia, placenta previa, loss of a twin, etc.

Knowledge is power, especially as an expectant Mother. The more you know and are informed, the easier it will be for you to navigate through your pregnancy and birthing experience in a deeply embodied way. We can learn from these stories to heal our timelines and create clear pathways for future generations of children to be born peacefully and for Mothers to feel safe, undisturbed and connected to their primal feminine wisdom.

Recode Your Birth Meditation

Find a comfortable position, sitting or lying down and gently close your eyes. Take a deep breath in and as you exhale, allow yourself to relax completely.

Begin by bringing your awareness to your breath. Feel your chest's gentle rise and fall with each inhale and exhale. Let each breath anchor you into the present moment.

Now visualise a warm, golden light surrounding you, enveloping you in a cocoon of safety and love. Feel this light permeating every cell of your being, filling you with peace and tranquillity. As you breathe deeply, imagine your mother appearing before you in whatever form feels most symbolic and comforting. Perhaps she appears as a radiant figure bathed in light or as a nurturing presence holding you in her arms. Whatever form she takes, know she is here supporting you on this journey.

TAKE a moment to connect with your mother's energy, feeling her love and presence surrounding you. Allow yourself to feel emotions, whether gratitude, forgiveness or simply a sense of connection. Now, bring your awareness to the moment of your birth. Visualise yourself being born into the world, surrounded by love and warmth. See yourself emerging into the world, pure and pristine, ready to embrace the journey ahead. As you witness your birth, allow yourself to feel deeply grateful for the gift of life. Know that you are a miracle, a precious being deserving of love and joy. Take a moment to bask in the beauty of your birth, feeling the love and support of your mother and the universe surrounding you. Know that you are cherished beyond measure.

Now, as you prepare to end your meditation, take a moment to thank your mother for the gift of life and the journey you have embarked upon together. Know that her love will always be with you, guiding you every step of the way. When you're ready, gently bring your awareness back to the present moment. Wiggle your fingers and toes, and slowly open your eyes. Remember, you are a divine being worthy of love and happiness. Carry the light of your birth within you always and know that you are deeply loved.

Take a moment to integrate, journal your thoughts and be present with the healing energy that wants to move through your body. It is possible to have a cathartic experience here, so be gentle with yourself and seek extra support if you need it.

Envisioning Your Motherhood Journey

Understanding the bigger picture at play here is important, ideally before you even begin your journey into pregnancy and birth. There is no guilt to carry if this is all new to you- it was to me, but when you know better, you do better... and when wisdom speaks, listen.

For the most part, our culture places a strong emphasis on pregnancy and birth as a physiological experience. When you understand the ripples that will be created from and through you, you can better prepare yourself for a beautiful pregnancy and Spiritual initiation into motherhood.

I want to say that this special time should be about creativity, sensuality, deep nourishment and gentle daily rhythms but I know that the pace of this modern world and the socio-political and economic stressors filter into our being whether we want them or not. By understanding how significant you are in the grand web of life, you can take your place knowing your responsibility, which is your ability to respond with strength and resilience. I hope this book stimulates your creativity in creating your own blueprint for motherhood so that you can carve your own path in alignment with the truth of your being, your capacity to truly love your children into maturity and to love your journey.

Motherhood is wildly messy and rewarding. It will stretch you in ways you've never experienced before. The best reminder I can offer to help you stay grounded and connected to the bigger dreaming at play is to remember that you are embarking upon the most sacred rite of passage and being initiated into the mother you are becoming.

I invite you to close your eyes and begin dreaming her in. Visualise her expressions in as much detail as possible. Let her be known to you. As you move through the pages of this book and find resonance, inspiration and insight, when there are moments of pause and stillness, place your hand on your heart and keep breathing her in.

You get to discover who you are as a mother, define her and allow that version of you to raise yourself- through all your wobbles, to embody her fully. You are in the initiation of becoming. Your wise self, the fully embodied mother and elder-Self is walking beside you every step of the way.

You're not alone.

4

SACRED RITES OF PASSAGE
UNDERSTANDING BIRTH AS A PROCESS OF INITIATION

> "Every rite of passage is an act of becoming, an act of taking responsibility for the self we are *choosing* to become. A meaningful rite weds knowledge to action, intention to expression, doing to being."
> -Abigail Brenne

As you journey through life from the innocence of infancy to the wisdom attained in elderhood, you traverse your timelines through a series of significant events, crossing the threshold from one state or identity into the next. These are known as *Sacred Rites of Passage*.

In many Indigenous and Neo-Pagan circles, these moments are revered and honoured with ritual and ceremony to mark transitions and personal initiations of profound significance. And now, amidst the hustle and bustle of the modern world, women are being called to reclaim the ancient wisdom and cyclic power of the womb by honouring their sacred rites of passage.

Through the Women's Mysteries, women across the world continue to explore the Divine Feminine, sharing stories, songs, mythology, symbology, feminine psychology, archetypal expressions and art whilst cultivating a sisterhood that celebrates the seasons of womanhood and the cycles of life, death and rebirth.

There are 4 main *Sacred Rites of Passage* specific to women, which signify potent transformation and initiation from one state of being into the next. These are blood rites and are as follows:

- *Birth (Universal)*
- **Menarche (Maiden)**
- **Sexual Initiation**
- **Pregnancy/Birth (Mother)**
- **Perimenopause/Menopause (Maga/Crone)**
- *Death (Universal)*

Each experience will shape your beliefs and perceptions of the world; they will define you and open you to new ways of viewing and expressing yourself. What is important to understand is that the energetic imprint of the first 3 initiations, Birth, Sexual Initiation and Menarche, can and will influence how you give birth.

Menarche

During Menarche, the womb 'comes online' for the first time and a young girl is initiated into Maidenhood through her first bleed. Please refer to my first book, Maiden. *A Mother's Guide to Puberty and Menarche as a Sacred Rite of Passage*[*] for the wisdom surrounding this season.

Sexual Initiation

Maidenhood lasts several years and shifts in expression upon sexual initiation. Sexual Initiation is significant as a rite of passage because it marks the transition from erotic innocence towards sexual maturity.

Through arousal, blood flows to the reproductive organs and in some cases, a woman will bleed upon penetration as the hymen stretches and tears. A young Maiden's energy field will shift once she has been pene-

---

[*] https://www.donnaraymond.com.au/courses/maidenbook

trated. If she is heterosexually oriented, she will need to map her cycle to guide her in understanding her hormonal and sexual impulses to be vigilant in safe sex practices and use contraception to avoid an unplanned pregnancy.

The first time a young woman engages in sexual activity, she will be imprinted with sensory information about her body, desires, pleasure, boundaries, sensuality, creativity and power. With sexual energy, it is important to note that arousal does not equate to consent, as the body can have a physiological response to external stimuli. This can cause a lot of confusion growing up, especially so considering the part of the brain that is responsible for cler rational thought does not fully develop until the aproximate age of 25.

It is necessary to consider what was playing out during this time of being initiated into the realms of sex, what was happening in your home life, the world and the community at large. Was it an empowering or disempowering experience?

Some questions to ask yourself that relate to your sexual initiation which may play out in the birth space:

- Did you feel respected?
- Did you feel in control?
- Were you listened to?
- Were your boundaries expressed and respected?
- Did it provide pleasure?
- Did you feel ready?
- Did you move at a pace that your body was ok with?
- Did you feel pressured or coerced?

Concerning sexual intercourse, it is also important to know that the energy of a partner can be unconsciously transferred into the womb. I started noticing this when I was in my late teens and discovered that I would start processing the unexpressed emotions of my partner days after we were physically intimate.

If there were suppressed emotions and discordant energy, I would begin to feel irritated, when I had no logical reason to be, or I would get a yeast infection. From an energetic perspective, the vagina is incredibly intelligent. She will tell you many things if you are willing to listen.

Sexual Trauma

When a woman is not ready in her body and Spirit to enthusiastically welcome and receive sexual energy and penetration into her inner world, she will harbour trauma, especially if she was a child at the time. These stories can then be hidden in shame and stored in the womb, sometimes carried for generations. I don't want to delve too deeply into the realms of sexual abuse and trauma, but it is important to know that a woman can heal from these imprints and reclaim her sovereign power over her body and inner domain.

This is delicate work and will need guidance from a professional who can help on all the levels required for deep healing. What I do need to express is that any stories about these experiences, the relationships involved, etc., will need to be looked at to clear the way for an empowered pregnancy and birth. During labour and birth, you will meet your edges, so there must be no stories blocking the way of you claiming dominion and safety over your own body, sexuality and innate power as a birthing woman.

On a side note, the visceral act of giving birth can be a big *'fuck you'* moment for many survivors and a reclamation of all that is sacred and fiercely holy.

A woman's initiation and journey through pregnancy and birth, as the Maiden meets herself as Mother, is incredibly powerful and sacred. The energetics of who you were during those initiations will appear at birth's doorstep as you transition from *Maiden to Mother*. That's why it is important to do the necessary 'inner work' of healing before you give birth. Ideally, you prepare yourself before you even conceive. Birth is an incredibly sexual experience, so if you have a history of abuse and trauma, you need to understand this so you can support yourself to feel empowered on your journey.

Birth as a Sacred Initiation

Rites of passage initiation rituals embody a sacred journey marked by distinct phases. They begin with separating from the familiar, followed by a transition characterised by symbolic trials, lessons and teachings. Initiates confront challenges that test their commitment and resolve, leading to a profound personal transformation. Ultimately, they reintegrate into their community with a renewed identity, fortified by symbolism of some kind and communal support.

Birthing a baby epitomises the pinnacle of *sacred rites of passage*, thrusting mothers into an enigmatic realm that grips their very being. Birth and death intertwine in a poignant dance, illustrating life's ephemeral beauty. Accepting birth necessitates embracing death as an intrinsic part of existence, a constant to be respected rather than feared. This paradox grants life a profound sacredness, shaping a continual evolution of bittersweet yet undeniably transformative growth.

I cannot emphasise enough the power of viewing birth as a language spoken through initiation and how it empowers and equips you to navigate the unknown with curiosity and wonder. A Mother is born anew with each birth, echoing ancestral legacies and epigenetic imprints. Lineage gains potency when rooted in identity and culture passed down through generations.

Birth is a portal to life and growth, with mothers undergoing physical and spiritual metamorphosis as they embark on the great work of labour and Matresence. Each birth is a unique dance, ushering mothers into Motherhood's sacred realm. However, the initiation of Maiden to Mother will leave women forever changed by the journey's profound depths of shifting identity and maturation.

With each consecutive pregnancy and birth, a woman is initiated into a depth of motherhood that she will be called to embrace and embody as she uncovers new versions of herself. Each initiation will require a sacrifice of the former version of herself. As she is reborn into her wisdom and power, she deepens into the busy season of Mother, guided by the Spirit and needs of each child and, of course, herself.

THE SEASON of Mother commands a level of maturity beyond the capacity seen in Maidenhood. An uninitiated Maiden, faced with the continuous demands of Mothering, will most likely cower at the magnitude of responsibility ahead. This internal struggle can lead to chaos as she grapples with unmet needs, triggering a cascade of stress responses.

Without the guidance of initiation, a Maiden thrust into Motherhood can cause much suffering and overwhelm as she battles for control, rebelling against the natural rhythms in a season that requires deep presence and surrender. This conflict between two competing energies can result in suffering and overwhelm, hindering her ability to surrender to the transformative power of Motherhood.

To avoid such turmoil, it's imperative for a Maiden to undergo her *sacred rite of passage* into her new identity as a fully embodied Mother. Through this initiation, she gains the wisdom and power necessary to navigate Motherhood with grace and confidence, embracing her maternal role and allowing her to channel her wild nature and sensual expression in a way that nurtures her psyche and ensures the vitality of future generations.

5

MAIDEN TO MOTHER
THE GREAT INITIATION

> "To be pregnant is to be vitally alive, thoroughly woman, and distressingly inhabitated. Soul and spirit are stretched- along with the body- making pregnancy a time of transition, growth, and profound beginnings."
> -Anne Christian Buchanan

The journey from *Maiden to Mother* is a profound spiritual initiation and sacred rite of passage, guiding women toward deeper maturity, wisdom, and creative power. It's a path open to all women, marking the transition from immature and youthful innocence to mature and responsible leadership. This initiation isn't solely about preparing for the physical act of giving birth, whether to a child or creative endeavours. It's a birthing of oneself as a mother and sovereign, a process of self-discovery and leadership.

Through this journey, women learn how to nurture and guide others and nurture and lead themselves, thereby shaping the world around them. It's a transformational journey of healing and empowerment where women embrace their roles as creators and caretakers with wisdom, grace and strength.

When a Maiden ventures into the realm of the Mother, she embarks on a profound journey that reshapes her on all levels. Motherhood, akin to navigating an ancient labyrinth, demands depths of presence and endurance beyond the reach of a Maiden. Though she may commence the journey, by design, she is fated to lose herself. Yet, by embracing the mystery and shedding preconceptions of self, she can ultimately find herself at the core, surrender herself in ritual and embrace her newfound responsibility as a mother with authenticity and purpose, making her way- spiralling out from the centre. This initiation serves as a necessary catharsis, stripping away solipsistic notions and birthing herself anew, revealing the truth of her essence as a sensual woman, creatrix and mother.

UNDERSTANDING this sacred initiation in three phases sheds light on the nonlinear nature of the journey, mirroring the wild, cyclical essence of nature itself. From pregnancy's encompassing journey to the singular physiological event of birth and onward through the continuous rebirth of motherhood, the spiral unwinds, and the 3 phases unfold:

1. **Separation:** A woman sheds her former identity, preparing to embrace motherhood. Physically and psychologically, she detaches from her previous life, allowing the mother archetype to emerge in her.
2. **Transition/Liminality:** In this liminal phase, uncertainty reigns as the woman prepares to give birth to a new life. Vulnerability and transformation mark this stage as she surrenders to her destiny, allowing a new existence to emerge.
3. **Integration:** Embracing her new identity as a mother, she reintegrates into society with her new roles and relationships. Rituals and ceremonies mark this phase, affirming her journey and solidifying her place in the community.

This process of initiation is not without pain and sacrifice as her body becomes a vessel for a new life and conscious awareness. From the demands of pregnancy to the intensity of childbirth and the mental and emotional load of motherhood, each stage presents its own trials, testing her endurance and resilience.

Pregnancy brings with it a flood of uncertainty, while childbirth itself is a deeply intense and visceral experience, pushing women to the edge of their fears and comfort. Emotionally, the transition is a whirlwind of conflicting thoughts and feelings, ranging from anticipation, excitement, joy, anxiety and vulnerability. After the birth, a new mother may grapple with hormone shifts and a spectrum of feelings, from overwhelming love to bone-tired exhaustion, accepting her postpartum body and identity within the home and community to the extreme ends of complete rejection and dissociation. She will move through moods of love and shame, celebration and self-doubt and the heavy realisation of how her life will continually shift to meet the growing demands, mental load and labour of raising a family and raising herself.

Spiritually, the journey into motherhood taps into the ancient and sacred essence of womanhood, aligning her with the timeless rhythms of creation. It awakens a profound sense of purpose and power as she nurtures new life and undergoes spiritual growth. Through this process, she gains insights into the interconnectedness of all living things, the mysteries of the womb and the ephemeral nature of life itself. Motherhood becomes her path to uncovering deep soul truths, fostering spiritual growth, patience, emotional resilience, healing and enriching the bond within herself, her child, and the world as she journeys toward maturity with grace, courage, and wisdom.

In essence, the initiation into motherhood is a multifaceted journey, weaving together physical, emotional and spiritual threads to form the tapestry of maternal wisdom and experience. Much of the journey is unknown. With unique threads that call her from the past into her ancestral stories and common threads that will weave through her story and help her connect with women around her, each woman will have her own initiatory experience and story to share.

Embracing the Maiden

Maiden, Mother, Maga, Crone. These powerful archetypal developmental stages relate to the seasons of a woman and the natural world. Each season of womanhood is marked by a change, which is intrinsically connected to the womb and the blood it gives in service to life, death and the natural world.

Maiden relates to spring and fertility and is entered through the portal of Menarche. Mother relates to the busy summertime and is entered through birthing. Maga relates to the autumn, a time of letting go and is initiated through peri-menopause. Crone is the winter, the time for deep roots and wisdom sharing as an elder, and it is entered via the portal of menopause and retirement, though nowadays, it is usually embodied in the later stages of life and relates to the power of legacy.

All of these seasons are imbued with energy and wisdom, which give meaning and context to our collective experience as women, though all of these seasons are imprinted with the power of the Maiden as she evolves through them into a seasoned, wise woman. It is through giving birth that the Maiden completely transforms as she bows in reverence at the feet of the Mother, who is just up ahead with arms wide open to take her hand and guide her to step into the great mystery, envelope her with self-love as she merges within and then they cross the threshold together, with mother at the helm.

The Gifts of the Maiden

Maiden energy is wild, curious and playful. She is open, fresh and wide-eyed with wonder. Her curiosity leads her down many paths without thought and her innocence and naivety mean she seeks world experiences in a more self-absorbed and hedonistic way. That is not to say it is a negative thing. Her awareness is more focused on developing an identity, exploring her desires and pleasures, her appearance, being liked by others and how she can move through the world freely. She is shaping her understanding of the world as she moves through it. Make no mistake, Maiden energy is also fierce, fiery, passionate, ungrounded and often destructive. Drama can be addictive. She can belong to no one until she belongs to herself.

MATURATION TAKES time to cultivate and unfortunately, our Western capitalist society only focuses on celebrating the sexually available aspects of the maiden. Her primal heat, beauty and sensuality have been commodified and weaponised, keeping many young women trapped in a cycle of abuse, materialism and emotional immaturity, which can, unfortunately, wreak havoc in their lives as they are transitioning into the season of Mother. By embracing the gifts of the Maiden, she can then merge with the Mother who wants to give birth through her.

Understand that you, as a woman, have multiple archetypal expressions that exist inside you at all times. It is vital that the Maiden transitions with the Mother as an integrated and whole-body expression. Any split within the psyche from an unintegrated expression will turn to shadow and may express in a distorted way, which in the realm of early motherhood can be akin to navigating a wild storm in the night with an inexperienced, rebellious teen at the helm. There's no right or wrong, only learning, so don't beat yourself up if you're reading this as a mature woman and you feel like you've missed something. Having this wisdom now will help you remedy choices that you've had to make in the past and help you reach back through time to heal parts of yourself that needed a wise hand to guide them.

MAIDEN ENERGY MUST BE ACKNOWLEDGED, expressed and embraced so she feels safe enough to embark on this sacred ego death and surrender into motherhood. This requires time, presence and ritual. It can not be rushed or forced; she will feel cornered and may rebel against the inner call to maturation.

Transitioning from Maiden to Mother does not mean you have to let this expression die. It simply means you integrate her playful and erotic innocence. She must willfully step aside and bow down to the altar of the Mother; in doing so, she claims her path to maturity, and Mother takes the lead. She must feel safe to embrace her transformation. This is how you step forward fully embodied and prepared for the journey ahead.

MOTHERHOOD IS a wild and sometimes turbulent journey of beautiful, messy growth. It requires patience, resilience and a sense of humour. Maiden energy can be too flighty to stay the course; she may try and trick herself into thinking that she is ready for the task at hand, but if unprepared, she will buckle under the pressure and demands of motherhood, especially in the modern world where we have lost connection to the support of the village and intergenerational living.

In the transition stages, you must cultivate a mindset conducive to growth and well-being on all levels. There is no point in doing any of this until you have addressed your subconscious beliefs about motherhood in general. That means looking at how you were mothered and the type of mother you aspire to be. This can be done before or during pregnancy and it is a priority to do so before birth.

JOURNALLING AND MEDITATION are easy ways to navigate your inner beliefs. Taking the time to sit in quiet introspection will help reveal what you value and what you don't. You will uncover beliefs that may shock you and are most likely not your own. You may find that you do not agree with some aspects of how you were raised and that will point you in the direction of how you choose to mother.

Grief may surface as you reflect on how you feel your inner child was truly seen or taken care of. You may begin to look at mothers you are inspired by, the role models that you want to emulate. All of this inner work will point you in the right direction to embodying your truth and provide the opportunity to clear the way of any residual beliefs and fears that keep you from accepting yourself as a mature, present, confident, loving mother.

If you feel stuck and need guidance, reach out for support in your community. You will most likely find many workshops and modalities in person and online. What you choose is up to you. The whole point is that you prioritise this work and treat this journey from *Maiden to Mother* as the sacred initiation that it is.

Integrating the Maiden

The journey from Maiden to Mother is one of the most important *Sacred Rites of Passage,* and we, as women, can walk it gracefully. If navigated consciously, the transition stages of late pregnancy can help women claim their role and responsibility as Mothers in a way that feels uplifting and inspiring.

I believe that when women walk through this sacred gateway with full commitment and presence, it helps to mitigate the risks of birth trauma and postpartum depression. Too many women have crossed the threshold of *Maiden to Mother* without a map and have lost themselves completely as the soul fragments into a suspended state of discombobulation. It is important to note that the map is not the territory, but it does help to make sense of what may lay ahead in the distance when you can't see or have the language to comprehend the magnitude of the journey into Motherhood. It's called the *Women's Mysteries* for a reason. You don't know what you don't know.

I HAVE SAT with many mothers in their darkness, I have witnessed heartache and pain, loss and longing, I have seen debilitating grief and suffering, deep soul pain, rage, doubt, resentment, frustration, loneliness and defeat. I've witnessed so much power and beauty in these raw human moments that I carry a torch to light up the dark with reverence and respect for the transformational cycles of birth, death and rebirth. There is nothing to fear, for you will only meet yourself in these spaces. Every birth will signify a metaphoric death of your identity as you know it, as the old makes way for the new. This is poetry in motion. This is Birth.

It is vital that you take the time to acknowledge this part of the passage and give yourself the time and space to reflect upon your journey up until the moment you cross that threshold into the vortex of Birth and Motherhood. This is done during the ripening stages of pregnancy by tapping into your creativity. If you are living life, you are creating every day. Perhaps that is creating a flourishing environment for your mental health and well-being. Express yourself in food, fibre, music, dance, somatic practices, writing, poetry, learning and storytelling, art, painting, drawing, collage, scrapbooking, nature walks, skating, swimming, reading books in random places, making memories, exploring fashion, colour texture, gardening, playing with reality, wearing odd socks or shoes simply because it delights you.

LET your Maiden energy be celebrated, and bring your full awareness to the freedom you have as a single-bodied woman! Your life is about to change in ways you can not comprehend from this state of being and to accept those changes fully, you will need to let go and grieve this version of yourself. Let yourself grieve, sister.

Let yourself sit with the enormity of what is taking place for you and inside of you. Make the time to connect with nature and your inner wisdom… feeling the ecstatic bliss of being alive, honouring your body as the divine vessel it is. Bring your awareness to the coming changes when one becomes two. Everything will rearrange. Expect it. Your world shifts to allow you to become the world for your baby.

THE ALCHEMY of Birth is that life as you know it will be completely transformed in unimaginable ways. You will be stretched beyond your perceived limits. Your child will help reveal parts of yourself you didn't know existed. You will experience strength, resilience, and love like you've never known. The egoic self will die a hundred deaths before your baby turns one. All relationships will be tested, especially intimate ones. So prepare to be humbled and grounded in the soulful service of Motherhood. Prepare to step into your power.

Integration Rituals

A ritual is a sequence of intentional activities or gestures that create spiritual meaning and significance for the participant. Rituals allow space for connection, reflection and reverence. By slowing down just a little, your ritual becomes a spiritual practice of mindfulness and helps you create and live a life rich with meaning and purpose.

Simple things are so often overlooked for their deep majick. Simple rituals like being in nature and feeling your heart swell with gratitude for being alive, freestyle movements and dance, somatic practices and singing help you to emotionally regulate and become more present with your life as it unfolds.

Brew your morning cuppa, and speak prayers and intentions into it. Write letters to express your emotions, and then burn them to release the weight you have been carrying. Journal your gratitude and reflect on who you are, where you've been and where you're going.

Words are spells, and our language helps us experience the world in particular ways. Majick exists in the mundane and is accessible to all who allow it into their lives. Energy flows where attention goes, so simple daily rituals will help you switch gears and become more present and anchored in life as it lives through you. Your presence is a gift to yourself and your loved ones.

Maiden Altar

An altar is an intentional space used for worship and devotional spiritual practices. They are used as a tool to 'alter' consciousness by the way you use and engage with it. Often, an altar will have specific symbolic items and tools relevant to its function. Keeping this in mind, you can start to think about what you'd like to create for a personal altar to honour your Maiden energy.

Begin by allocating a sacred space to create a Maiden altar. This will be a special area that has significance for you to begin the integration process and for those of you who are reading this and are in the depth of motherhood and feel lost, this will help you revive your Spirit and reclaim parts of yourself that have been cast into the shadow. I recommend placing your altar in an area that is out of the way of your daily activities, yet still a part of your daily life.

Think about how you would like to interact and use your altar and the rituals you will create. If you're more prone to inner reflective work like journalling and meditation, you won't require as much floor space around your altar as if you were to dance or engage in somatic practices. Think about the area you need to set up and allow your intuition to guide you in its creation. If you're being called to create an altar out in nature, do so. If it's on a shelf inside, go with it! Follow your inner guidance. This is not something you can get wrong.

Trust yourself. If you want to give birth at home, consider setting up the altar in your birth space. Once you move through the emotional and spiritual integration of Maiden, you can adapt and redefine your altar to activate the birth field and acknowledge your new identity as a mother.

As you create your Maiden altar, start collecting and displaying photographs or personal items (things like letters, toys, jewellery, trinkets, crystals, ticket stubs and wrist bands, music, art, etc) that remind you of your wild, playful nature, your rebelliousness, your childlike innocence. All expressions of Maiden energy are welcome here, especially if your teenage years were reckless or traumatic. Create a space for all parts of yourself to be seen, welcome and loved. This is about calling yourself home- to yourself.

Spend a few days or weeks collecting objects that beautify the space and hold deep meaning and significance. If you are taking anything from Nature, you must ask permission first, make sure you have a clear yes and then give something back to the land you gather from. Do not remove rock from any waterways. Not only are they sacred, but they are also an important part of the ecosystem, waterways and natural habitats for insects. As a general rule, try to collect things with minimal disturbance to the landscape.

If you follow religious or majickal practices, you may like to include symbolism in your altar to amplify its spiritual energy. Consider objects that represent the elements and speak to the power of creation. Once your altar is complete, place a candle in the centre to draw the energy inwards and light it when you begin your daily rituals of connection and integration.

Interact with this altar daily. Sing, dance, journal and meditate in a way that consciously connects to your Maiden energy. Let your Maiden energy guide you towards what she wants and needs so that she feels seen, heard and held in her fullness.

Meditation

Sit quietly with your eyes closed and begin to focus on your breath. Breathe slowly and rhythmically, drawing your awareness and breath into the womb. Keep breathing until you feel connected to your body. Take as long as you need.

Visualise your Maiden self standing before you when you feel present and grounded. This may be you as you are now, or it may be a few years younger. Allow 'her' to present herself to you freely. This may take some time- it may take several attempts, particularly if you have experienced trauma and dissociation.

Be gentle with yourself and be present. You are not here to go into any story or pain; simply bring your awareness to who she is and her core-essence.

Allow yourself to receive her beauty, innocence and power in this moment. Meet her from the perspective and embodiment of the Mother... as if she were your child. Look at her with love, adoration and fondness. Stay in this moment of connection for as long as you can and allow the dynamic of Maiden and Mother to exchange energy in whatever way it moves through you.

If your Maiden is very reserved or feels far away, you may like to keep returning to this mediation over several days to create a sense of safety so she may reveal herself to you. You are building a relationship here. Again, be gentle with yourself and be present with what is. You (in your Mother state) may wish to speak words of life into her that help her light up, honouring and valuing who she is unconditionally. Speak the words you would have longed to hear. Speak life into yourself. Allow yourself to Mother yourself.

Visualise yourself embracing the Maiden and celebrate her! Offer gratitude for how far she has travelled to get here, to this moment. Honour her courage and Spirit. During this part, you may feel her morph into you or see her standing before you and stepping into you... as if you merge and become one. However this plays out, the purpose is to create a visual or somatic experience of integration that she is not getting left behind because she is coming with you!

Alternatively, you may also like to create a similar journey from the perspective of embodying your Maiden and meeting your Mother energy for the first time... then stepping into her. Do what is right for you. When you finish your integration meditation, sit quietly and stay with your breath. Be in the moment.

Start to bring gentle movement to your body before opening your eyes, and then journal or voice record your experience if it feels right.

Journal Prompts

- In what ways do you express yourself creatively?
- What type of attention does your Maiden energy crave?
- What does she do if she doesn't receive it?
- What does your Maiden energy need from you to feel safe, seen and held?
- What does she need you to know?
- What forgiveness does she need to give that anchors her to the past?
- What lights your Maiden energy up, and how will this need to change and evolve as you become a Mother?
- What big projects do you want to create in this lifetime?
- What beliefs do you have about Motherhood?
- What does being a Mother mean to you?
- How will you connect with your self-identity and purpose before and after becoming a Mother? How do you think this will change? What is non-negotiable?
- What qualities of mothering are you inspired by and why?
- What role models do you have, and what do you love about them?
- Why is that important to you?
- What do you feel your mother got right in how she raised you?
- What qualities/skills/beliefs do you want to pass on to your child?
- In what ways could the way your mother parented you improve?
- What fears or worries do you have about being a Mother?

- Are you able to learn or figure out any of these skills?
- Who is in your support network? How can you create one now?
- What do you need from your partner to feel safe, secure and supported on this journey?
- What do you wish they knew but you're afraid to tell them?
- What are your thoughts on losing yourself or your relationship in the role of Mother? How can you remedy this?
- What do you want your children to think of when they reflect on their childhood?
- What do you wish you had done before becoming a Mother?
- If they feel important to you, can you live with putting those things on hold for a while, or will you regret it?
- If you were to die during childbirth, what type of life would you hope for your child, and who would that be with?
- What would you want them to implement on your behalf?
- How do you envision your pregnancy?
- What type of birthing experience would you like to have?
- How do you see your postpartum time? Who are your support people?
- How can you and your partner prioritise time together in the chaos of child-rearing?
- What are your non-negotiable that will foster connection, intimacy and teamwork?

PART II- PREPARATION
NURTURING THE SPIRITUAL CONNECTION DURING PREGNANCY

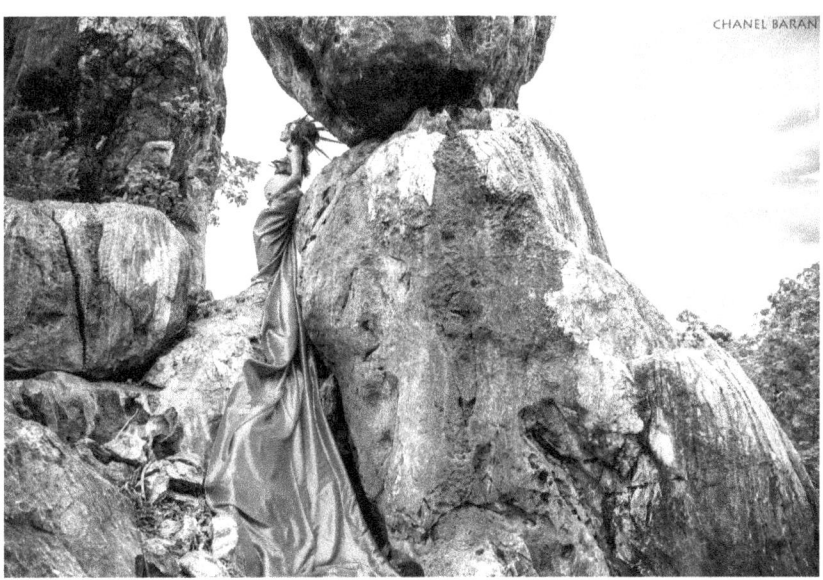

"For far too many women pregnancy and birth is something that happens to them rather than something they set out consciously and joyfully to do themselves." -Sheila Kitzinger

6

CONCEPTION
CONSCIOUS CO-CREATION

"We create a New Earth from the place within us that is pure positive energy wanting to give and receive love. It is time to awaken from the unconscious sleeping and live in the conscious dreaming."
-Betty Lenora

Physiologically speaking, conception happens at the moment sperm meets a fertile egg. On average, a man ejaculates between 2-5ml of semen, which contains around 20 million sperm per ml; around 1,000 make it into the fallopian tubes, and only 1 will fertilise an egg. The vagina and the womb are quite hostile environments for sperm, but once they reach the fallopian tubes, the sperm follow a chemical signal secreted by the fertile egg.

During the average woman's menstrual cycle, there are six days when intercourse can result in pregnancy; this 'fertile window' comprises the five days before ovulation and the day of ovulation itself. Just as the day of ovulation varies from cycle to cycle, so does the timing of the six fertile days. Cervical mucus helps sperm live up to 5 days in a woman's body, and it takes around 6 hours for active sperm to reach the fallopian tubes.

. . .

THE 2020 STUDY TITLED: *Chemical Signals from Eggs Facilitate Cryptic Female Choice in Humans*[1], challenges the traditional belief that the fastest sperm wins. Instead, it suggests that the egg plays an active role by releasing chemical signals and follicular fluid that assist in selecting the most desirable sperm based on the quality of the genetic material encoded within. This concept of *'cryptic choice'* echoes the spiritual sentiments of the feminine opening and receiving the masculine rather than being forced by penetration. In this way, conception is not an act of violence but rather a powerful dance and sacred union.

An egg, once released, is only viable for 12-24 hours, though sperm can live inside the vagina for up to 5 days. During ovulation, the female ovaries will produce progesterone, which promotes pregnancy by thickening the tissues of the womb wall. Once the sperm has been granted entry into the egg, a complex chain of events begins to take place and a fertilisation window spans approximately 15-16 hours. During this time, cells begin to divide as the genetic codes from the sperm and egg merge into the centre of the egg. This union of cells is called a zygote and evolves to form the developing embryo. Between days 4 and 6, after fertilisation, known as the blastocyst stage, fluid starts to fill inside the embryo, the outer cell walls develop, and the inner cells begin to form a baby.

A few days later, the blastocyst will cascade down from the fallopian tubes and eventually implant itself into the womb wall. This is a crucial stage of pregnancy, as the embryo connects with the Mother by sending chemical signals into the bloodstream to continue producing progesterone to support and help the embryo develop into a baby. Pregnancy is obtained once everything is in perfect and Divine order; sperm reaching the egg, temperature, genetic material matching, cells dividing, and implantation happens correctly. If less than ideal, the Mother's body may perceive this new embryo as a foreign contaminant and reject it, resulting in termination of pregnancy, what we call miscarriage, which usually takes place in the first 12 weeks but can occur naturally up to 20 weeks of pregnancy.

Dr Roger Pierson, director of the reproductive biology research unit at the University of Saskatchewan, said that in a recent study, it was noted that 40% of female subjects had the potential to produce more than one egg in a single month. Out of the 68 participants- 6 ovulated twice.[2] This is not a new concept, it is quite ancient.

Cosmic Connections

In ancient mythology, the moon was revered as the embodiment of female power and the Mother Goddess. Often linked with fertility, the moon was closely associated with the growth of plants and trees. Its changing phases, from crescent to full, symbolised birth and death; while its role as the giver of rain underscored its connection to fertility. Ancients believed that just as the moon influenced plant fertility, it also played a crucial role in the fertility of animals.

In 1956, Dr. Eugene Jonas, a Czechoslovakian Psychiatrist and Astrologer, discovered the *Lunar Fertility Method* from an ancient Babylonian text. This method, known today as the *Jonas Method,* blends astrology with conception timing, considering moon phases and a woman's astrological sign at birth. It proposes that a woman's fertility is influenced by her physiological cycle and cosmic and astrological cycles governed by the moon and the sun. Jonas's research revealed that a woman's fertility correlates with the moon phase at birth, allowing for spontaneous ovulation and multiple monthly chances of conception. Moreover, the moon's astrological position and sign may influence the baby's gender, while specific gravitational forces can impact pregnancy. The female body continues to hold many mysteries.

Co Creation

Conscious Co-Creation happens when, by rite, mother and father journey in sacred union together to dream in the Spirit of their child and either make love with the pure intention to conceive in that exchange or are at peace with the possibility of conception via their union, surrendering to an organic timeline of pregnancy.

Sexual energy is one of the most potent energies on the planet; it is the most you can merge with a person physically, and when channelled for the pure purpose it has been designed for, the template of the incarnating child is imbued with the energy of this love and connection.

Having said that, the Spirit of a child can visit parents independently. Thus, two souls hook into the *'dream seed'*. Spirit weaves majick to align those parents with procreating a child, sometimes not necessarily to be partners or parents together, but for the sheer genetic and limbic imprinting needed for a soul's evolution. I'm not saying this is ideal, though it sure makes sense spiritually and can explain a lot of modern relating.

Conscious Conception- Dreamseeds

In a spiritual context, conception happens when the mother or father conceives a child in *The Dreaming*. What I mean by *The Dreaming* is the infinite potential of creation energy and consciousness, the realm where all possibilities and timelines co-exist in Divine beauty and harmony.

Spiritually speaking, when the child's soul meets the parent, a spark of light is created in the etheric dimension, and a contract is created in the heart with a blueprint of how that Soul chooses to come through. If conditions are ripe and the timeline is in sync, the new soul will have a clear pathway for incarnation into the physical world. So, you may have found yourself dreaming of a child many years before the actual physical conception.

All of my children were *dream seeds*. It's as if our souls met and made a plan together. When I was 18, my firstborn, Auraura Freedom, came through strongly in this way. I write more about that experience in the *Sacred Birth Stories* section at the end of this book, where I share all of my birth stories.

I've always trusted that I am connected to something bigger, a Divine intelligence that orchestrates synchronicities that help guide me to my ultimate destiny and purpose in this lifetime. Call it God's plan, if you prefer.

Following this path and trusting the process has proven to be incredibly rewarding, even if, at the time, I do not completely understand the meaning behind why certain things play out the way they do. What is interesting to note is that upon my surrender to the divine plan and wisdom of her knowing, she left my energetic field and didn't return until 2 years later when I met her father, and in an instant, I knew he was the 'one'. Not as a life partner but as Auraura's chosen father, undoubtedly.

Karmic Entanglement

Karma is a Sanskrit word that means 'action' or 'doing' and relates to the universal lore of cause and effect. It is neither good nor bad. It simply allows the experience for an individual to be responsible for their life and choices.

Sometimes, conception happens under the confines of a karmic entanglement, whereby the parents are locked into a karmic relationship, a soul tie, contract or debt from a former timeline, which plays out in this realm, resulting in the birth of a child or children. Usually, these karmic relationships do not work out in the long run because the purpose of the union was to create a new soul into being, in agreement to facilitate the soul's path of evolution.

All relationships in this entanglement are to perpetuate mutual growth and evolution on a Soul level. There can be very complex relationship dynamics at play. As well as you think you've planned your life path or done things the 'right' way according to your society, karmic relationships will reveal themselves in time as the truth comes to light. It is important to note that no matter your circumstances or how your life unfolds, acceptance and forgiveness are necessary on your path as a conscious parent. It's important to do the necessary healing work so you don't project unhealed wounds from the relationship onto your child. Unless there was abuse at play, your child has a right to create meaningful connections with their other parent, regardless of how you feel about them. Have enough respect for your child's development to keep the adult stuff to adults.

Preparing the Soul Soil

To create the optimum environment for conscious conception, it is wise for both parents to prepare themselves for the journey before physical conception. Ideally, this means cultivating a strong sense of intimacy as a couple, connecting with your soul purpose, cultivating emotional resilience and healing ancestral/childhood traumas while preparing the body. For a male, this means preparing his seed. Semen, in essence, is a map of genetic material to be passed on to create new life. For a woman, it means preparing the soil- her womb, for which the seed will take root.

Suppose a couple works together with the same intention to conceive. In that case, the energy around them is amplified and providing no medical reasons why conception can not take place, the miracle of creation can bless them both in incredible ways that provide profound personal growth. Working on a positive and uplifting mindset will help to raise the body's vibration, thus transmitting a frequency that calls to the inspired potential of consciousness yearning to experience itself through you.

Some practices that help with preparing the fertile "*soul soil*" for conception are:

- Journaling
- Embodiment practices
- Meditation
- A diet of whole and living foods
- Creative expression- art, music, dance
- Mindset work
- Dreaming
- Transformational healing
- Connecting with Nature
- Sitting with and seeking counsel from elders
- Deepening into your spiritual practice
- Emotional alchemy
- Community connections.
- Digital Detox

Another key element for preparation is actively inviting your child's energy into your space. If you find that you decorate things in pairs, begin to add a third to the mix. Look at your home and take note of the energy you are surrounded by. Does your home feel fertile, exuding a welcoming energy for a child, or does it feel bland and sterile?

Caress your wombspace as if your child already resides there; this powerful symbolic gesture calls to your child's Spirit. With all my children, I found myself intuitively caressing my belly as if I was pregnant before I had conceived. This is another way I knew a baby was in my field and wanted to come through the portal of my womb.

As a couple, bringing playful energy into your discussions about conceiving and raising a child is extremely beneficial. It is important to share similar values for raising your child and discuss the real and practical side of the emotional, physical and financial roles and responsibilities of raising a child. How will you both prepare for the inevitable disruption of your lifestyle that a new baby brings?

Creating space for this vulnerable openness fosters intimacy and trust, making safety and minimising stress. Finding solutions to potential problems before you conceive can lift the weight of subconscious fears and insecurities that may be blocking you both energetically from conceiving in the first place. This is also true for the duration of pregnancy. This type of maturity and 'real talk' is vital for healthy and thriving relationships, whether as a couple or as co-parents.

Women give birth to children, just as the Earth offers life to plants. Women feed the children, and the Earth does the same. The majick of women is the majick of the Earth. The womb is the soil where dreamseeds take root, bud and blossom to birth. The power that creates and feeds is truly a feminine force.

The Importance of Womb Work

As a woman, it is important to connect with the inherent power of the womb, not only to deepen into your embodied presence and radiance, but to also check-in and 'clean house' of any tension or residual emotional debris that becomes stored in the body. This is especially important pre-conception, though it can be facilitated effectively and safely throughout pregnancy. One of the most powerful ways I know to do this is via my emotional alchemy practice, WombSong. *

---

* Raymond, D. (2015) *WombSong Emotional Alchemy Practice: A Transformational Journey*

I have had many women come to my *WombSong* workshops and use my online course, which has helped with releasing deep-seated fears, anger, rage, frustration, grief, and guilt, clearing their wombspace of heavy energy, and within months, conceiving.

I do not promote this as a definitive tool for pregnancy because every woman has a different experience. With the rise of modern infertility, there is no way I could ever purport that *WombSong* will result in pregnancy because there are enough modalities that prey upon women's vulnerabilities and I refuse to operate on that level.

What I do promote and know from experience is that women who engage in womb work, like *WombSong,* have a deeper connection to their body, beauty and intuition, engage in the world in a more present and receptive way and carry less stress and tension with them day to day. Womb Work helps women claim their sovereignty as fully embodied, sensual women, which is incredible in and of itself. However, when preparing to become a Mother, it is such a gift to be able to offer our children.

Due to the effects of limbic imprinting, I feel that women must energetically prepare the wombspace to create an environment that fosters health, vitality, joy, beauty and abundance. Cleaning the house before the new tenant arrives so to speak!

Soul Song

I received a song when I connected with the Spirit of my babies. Each one had a unique melody and came through at different stages during pregnancy. When you allow yourself to drop into the deepest presence, you can listen intently to the whispers of your child in Spirit or utero. The *soul song* is another form of conception that helps anchor the child into the physical world.

Once the song has come through, you can sing this unique tune to your developing child. This becomes a songline for the baby to track,

---

Towards Emotional Liberation, Creative Sensual Expression and Awakening Your Sacred Feminine Wisdom, [online course], Available at: https://www.donnaraymond.com.au/courses/womb song encoding the land with the energetic imprint of the new soul. It offers a sense of belonging and comfort. Once the baby is earthside, this song can be a soothing remedy to settle a distressed and overstimulated newborn. The song becomes a way to connect one's Spirit to the protection of the womb, where everything is familiar and safe.

Overall, it is important to see conception beyond the physical act of sexual reproduction. It is much more vast and nuanced than this limited way of thinking and perceiving.

Dream Seed Meditation

Several years ago, I created a powerful seed meditation, and I'd love to share it with you for free. **donnaraymond.com.au/dreamseedmeditation.***

---

* *I suggest you return to this meditation after you finish reading the book, as you will gain more powerful insights along the way, which will help you connect with your creative energy.*

7

SACRED PREGNANCY

MYSTICAL MATERNITY AND ACTIVATING THE WOMB GRID

> "My body, my life, became the landscape of my son's life. I am no longer merely a thing living in the world;
> I am a world."
> *-Sarah Manguso*

The Womb is sacred and powerful. All human life generates inside this creative vortex and births us all through the eyes of the *Great Mystery*. Pulsing with majick and potential, of playful sensual nature and power, the womb comes online through a blood offering and sacrament to the *Divine Feminine* in flow... ebbing with the changing seasons of life and death. Renewing and remembering.

Pregnancy is a time of profound connection, growing life consciously, which is a deeply physical experience as much as spiritual. The more you bring your awareness and presence into these physical sensations, the more connected you feel to your body, baby and the timeless wisdom surrounding pregnancy and birth. Many lessons are offered through the portal of pregnancy as your body shifts and changes to accommodate the birth of a new being. For some women, pregnancy feels incredibly easy and for others, the journey is hard and complicated. Your experience of pregnancy does not equate to your success or failure as a woman. It is a personal journey and exploration of sensations in the *Soma*- the body.

There are four different types of pregnancy that women can experience.

- **INTRAUTERINE PREGNANCY (NORMAL PREGNANCY)** A normal pregnancy develops favourably when the embryo correctly implants into the lining of the uterus.
- **MULTIPLE PREGNANCY.** Two or more eggs are fertilised by two or more sperm (fraternal twins or multiples), or when the zygote splits at an early developmental stage leading to identical twins.
- **ECTOPIC PREGNANCY (EXTRAUTERINE)** The embryo implants and grows outside the uterus. There are different locations in the female reproductive tract where this can happen, mainly in the fallopian tubes and less commonly in the abdominal cavity or the cervix.
- **MOLAR PREGNANCY**- The egg is incorrectly fertilised, and the placenta develops abnormally, forming various cysts.

You will be stretched to your full capacity as your womb swells with life. From the earliest stages of conception to the moment of birth, fetal development is a testament to the marvels of life and the intricate dance of nature unfolding within the womb. Tracking this development week to week- can help you focus your attention and channel your energy into connecting with the growth of those cells and organs- especially if you're having a tough pregnancy due to things like hyperemesis gravidarum, placenta previa, preeclampsia, gestational diabetes, mental health and sensory overwhelm, premature rupture of membranes or any other health conditions that make it difficult to naturally feel connected to the beauty of birth and your changing body.

There are several online maternity mailing lists you can join, which will ask you to enter your last known period (LNP) or conception dates so that you can receive weekly development emails to track your baby's growth. This is a wonderful resource to help visualise and focus your energy on your growing baby. Here's a simplified version.

Week 1-4: First Trimester, Conception to Implantation

- Conception occurs when sperm fertilises the egg, forming a zygote. The zygote undergoes rapid cell division, forming a blastocyst.
- Around day 6-7, the blastocyst implants into the uterine lining.
- The placenta begins to develop, providing nutrients and oxygen to the growing embryo.

Week 5-8: Embryonic Period

- The embryo undergoes rapid growth and differentiation.
- Organs and body systems, including the neural tube (which develops into the brain and spinal cord), heart, lungs, digestive system and limbs, begin to form.
- Facial features like eyes, ears and nose start to take shape.
- The embryo is called a foetus by the end of the embryonic period.

Week 9-12: Second Trimester

- The foetus continues to grow rapidly, doubling in size during this period.
- External genitalia begin to differentiate, although sex cannot yet be determined via ultrasound.
- Fingers and toes become more defined and nails begin to form. Facial features become more distinct, and the foetus may start to make involuntary movements.

Week 13-16

- The foetus continues to grow and develop, with the head becoming more proportional to the body.

- Muscles and bones continue to develop and the foetus may begin to move more actively.
- Facial expressions, such as frowning and squinting, may be observed via ultrasound.
- The digestive system starts producing meconium, the baby's first bowel movement, accumulating in the intestines.

Week 17-20

- The foetus undergoes a growth spurt, with significant weight gain and increased muscle mass.
- Lanugo (fine hair) covers the body, helping to regulate body temperature.
- Vernix caseosa, a thick waxy substance, covers the skin to protect it from amniotic fluid.
- The fetal heartbeat may be audible with a stethoscope.
- Movement becomes more coordinated, and the mother may feel fluttering sensations (quickening).

Week 21-24

- The foetus grows and develops, with the skin becoming less transparent.
- Eyebrows and eyelashes develop, and the eyes begin to open.
- The lungs continue to mature, with alveoli (air sacs) forming.
- Taste buds develop on the tongue, and the foetus may swallow amniotic fluid.
- Brain development accelerates with increased neuronal connections and activity.

Week 25-28: Third Trimester

- The foetus's body becomes more proportionate, increasing fat deposits for insulation and energy storage.
- Lung development continues, with surfactant production increasing to aid in breathing.

- The baby may start to hiccup.
- The foetus's sensory organs, including vision, hearing, taste and touch, become more developed.
- The foetus may respond to external stimuli, such as light and sound, with movements or changes in heart rate.
- The brain undergoes rapid growth and development, with increasing complexity and functionality.

Week 29-32

- The foetus continues to gain weight rapidly, with the body filling out and becoming more rounded.
- Rapid eye movements (REM) may be observed during sleep cycles.
- The bones continue to harden, although the skull remains soft and flexible to facilitate passage through the birth canal.
- The foetus may assume a head-down position in preparation for birth.
- Maturation of the central nervous system allows for more coordinated movements and reflexes.
- If the baby is born during this period, it will be classed as 'preterm'.

Week 33-36

- The foetus's growth slows as it approaches full term, with most major organs and systems fully developed.
- The lungs continue to mature, with surfactant production increasing to facilitate breathing after birth.
- The foetus's skin becomes smoother as fat deposits increase under the skin.
- The foetus may settle into a head-down position in the pelvis in preparation for birth.
- The Mother may experience more frequent Braxton Hicks contractions as the uterus prepares for labour.

Week 36-40: Full Term

- The foetus is considered full-term and ready for birth.
- The foetus grows and gains weight, although growth may slow in the final weeks.
- The foetal head may engage in the pelvis in preparation for labour.
- The Mother may experience signs of impending labour, such as the onset of regular contractions, cervical dilation and the release of the mucus plug.
- The average length of pregnancy is around 40 weeks, although labour may occur anytime between 37 and 42 weeks gestation.

Meaningful Maternity

Now is the time to nurture yourself as your body works over time. You may feel energetically depleted, so focus on healthy nutrition, prioritising rest, relaxation and reducing stress. If you think about it, you are not afforded many opportunities in this lifetime to have this experience. Savour it. This miracle of life, nestled in your womb and the transformations inside your body can be akin to a spiritual awakening. Meaning is created through presence, connection and your ability to find the majick in the mundane. The meanings you assign to what you experience daily can shape your lived reality and how you move through life. Be mindful of the stories you tell yourself and be open to unlearning what has been modelled to you. Each trimester will bring a different energetic imprint and if you are present enough, you will catch some powerful yet subtle shifts and insights.

First Trimester

I do not recommend announcing your pregnancy publicly until after the initial 12 weeks, as this means you have a higher chance of a viable pregnancy. Start taking photos of your changing body as a keepsake. During my *Maiden to Mother* journey, I purchased a disposable camera and took a side-on photo every week to see my body in bloom. They are among some of my most cherished photos and have created powerful portals for healing, which I didn't know at the time I would need in the future.

Documenting the growth of your growing womb and journaling your thoughts and feelings will help you connect with your wombspace, your child's Spirit and the mystical side of maternity. The words you write may help your child's self-development journey later in life, if and when they start to unpack their *origin story* and *limbic imprint*. It can be a beautiful time if you allow it- provided your body responds well to pregnancy. Encourage your partner (If you have one) to connect with you so that they may also be witness to the changes.

START THINKING about the months ahead and how you can optimise the energy of your pregnancy to reach your desired goals. Consider what your life will be like when you are called to slow down. What can you do now to support that? What plans can you implement, and what resources can be set aside? Never underestimate what you can get done in such a short amount of time. Pregnancy has a funny way of narrowing your focus and investing your energy into things that truly matter long-term.

Your pregnancy is not a limitation. It is an invitation to prioritise where you focus and share your energy. For the most part, it is more of an inwards journey, but if you're a prolific creator- you will do just that! I started painting, began my entrepreneurial journey, ran my first *Womb-Song* workshop and 4-day transformational healing retreat, birthed the *Wise Wombman Mystery School* and *Sacred Circles facilitator training*[*], started writing this book and more- all while pregnant with one of my children.

If there are creative ideas and projects that you've been procrastinating on, it's a good time to fire up your motivation to get stuff done before the demands of motherhood kick in. No matter how much you plan, that newborn stage will kick you in the arse at some stage so that you come off your high horse and ground you back down to Earth.

---

[*] https://www.donnaraymond.com.au/courses/sacred-circle-sisterhood

It is important to note that *all pregnancies result in birth* and should be honoured and treated as such. If you are choosing to not continue your pregnancy through to term, honour your no as soon as possible. Before 7 weeks gestation is ideal and will allow for an easier medical miscarriage, emotionally, spiritually and physically. In Buddhism, the soul is held for 49 days between death and rebirth. If you experience a spontaneous miscarriage during this time, seek help to process your loss and the support you need to integrate the experience and nurture yourself during your postpartum journey.

Journaling your thoughts and experiences will become sacred and valuable to you as you look back on this window of time. Be present with life as it unfolds. Be conscious of your energy and your thoughts. I share more on this in the Sacred Spiral chapter.

Recap- First Trimester lessons:
Be with what is, without force.
Adjust your decisions and actions accordingly.
Connect with and nourish your changing body.
Get started on your creative projects

Second Trimester

From around 5 months gestation, slow down and connect with the baby more deeply. Find at least one activity that fills your cup and focus on your creativity. All the things you have postponed in the past, start exploring those passions now. Create more intimacy with your partner if you have one, learn a new instrument, create art, dance, learn, explore and work with a mentor. The more you invest in nurturing your soul's inspiration, creativity and passions, the more you will deeply connect with your child and imprint it with the energy of creativity and vitality.

Every day, walk barefoot on country (on the land) and connect with the *Great Mother*. Of course, this is relative to the seasons and your situation. If you're stuck indoors, consider creating an Earthy altar. Connecting with the primordial mother energy and the natural world will help to reduce stress, anxiety and worry.

Connect with other mothers, join or host a women's circle (I can teach you how to do that) and listen to positive and uplifting birth stories. Protect your space, both physically and emotionally. This will be a time for you to exercise and vocalise your boundaries, as suddenly, you'll be surrounded by 'experts' with a plethora of unsolicited advice and fearful stories. You are under no obligation to expose yourself to madness.

As your pregnancy progresses, you may feel the flutters of movement in your womb called *the quickening*. This may bring up some emotion as suddenly things become real. Be with it. Your Maiden energy may want to reject and rebel against the changes happening. Allow her the space to react safely so that your inner Mother can respond to her with gentle, loving presence and guidance. Ego deaths do not need to be painful and can be a fabulously wild and humbling journey if met with curiosity and wonder as opposed to pressure, guilt and shame.

Take advantage of growth hormones; your hair and nails will be supercharged and lustrous. You may also feel an increase in erotic energy and arousal. Explore this and celebrate your sexuality and feminine pleasure unashamedly. Find ways to play and be out in the world. Be mindful of limbic imprinting. Avoid dramatic social situations and above all else, seek ways to protect your peace.

RECAP- SECOND TRIMESTER LESSONS:
Slow down.
Protect your peace.
Support and nourish your body and your creativity.
Embrace your erotic energy and pleasure.
Allow your inner Mother to hold space for the Maiden to express herself unashamedly- so that she may be integrated fully before the birth of your baby

Third Trimester

The third trimester is the time to advocate for yourself. Engage and speak to your birth support team, partner, doula, midwife and doctors. If you've chosen to give birth in a hospital setting, you may be able to visit the birthing suites to start familiarising yourself with the environment and hospital protocols. Ask questions! My first midwife, Gabrielle, shared this prompt to help me navigate the lead-up to birth,

> "What's it for, and is it necessary?"

This helps to foster autonomy and informed consent for birthing women when dealing with the medical establishment when it feels like they want to poke, prod and coerce you. You have to advocate for yourself and speak up from a place of inner authority.

If you have elected to have a cesarean, consider having a conversation with your obstetrician to see if they are open to the practice of *gentle cesarean*, which mimics the slow emergence of natural birth, with immediate, prolonged skin-to-skin contact and delayed cord clamping.

These last few months of pregnancy are a call to clear the way for a positive birth experience. This means having the necessary conversations with your partner, birth support team and any medical professionals you've engaged for care during your upcoming birth.

Begin to explore all the ways you can become a *Birth Warrior* and create peace and safety around you that will support you in a beautiful birthing journey. If you're birthing at home, begin to designate your space and claim it energetically, having it all set up early may not be practical. Still, you can begin to engage with the space, sing, dance, light candles and practice your rituals to activate the *birth field*. The more you become comfortable in the space you have chosen to birth, the easier it will be for you to surrender during labour. Practice your emotional alchemy and shadow work in this space, but avoid heavy energy like arguments.

During these last weeks, you will begin to open up energetically into the *birth field*. If you're sensitive to energy, you will feel the subtle shift. You will feel the pull to soften and slow down. You will feel like you are being called inwards and naturally withdraw yourself from external sensory stimulation and activities. You may start to receive deep wisdom from within your womb as your baby takes up more space, pushing out what you may need to face and come to peace with before the journey and initiation of birthing. Your dreams may become even more lucid and intense, and you may also start to receive wisdom and spiritual insights about your gifts and purpose beyond mothering. Listen.

I suggest that, from 33 weeks onwards, you disconnect from the synthetic machine world. If you want to give birth unassisted, I would completely switch off and disconnect from the external stimulus completely, from 35 weeks. This will provide adequate time to 'drop in' and be completely present with your day's natural rhythm and flow and help you awaken to your sensual nature as a fertile woman, ripe with creation. Creating time for stillness will help you prepare emotionally and spiritually for the journey ahead. You will get a surge of energy known as *nesting* which tells you you are ripening.

There is also an innate erotic energy that you can tap into and harness, which helps to stimulate oxytocin. Embrace your sexual energy if it is present in your body. Make love and art. It is an exquisite special experience to feel so fully ripe and erotically alive in your body.* The energy is palpable. This is the perfect time to book a maternity photoshoot to celebrate your beautiful, lusciously full body!

Recap- Third Trimester lessons:

Communicate your wants, needs and desires with your birth team as clearly and succinctly as possible so that everyone is on the same page.

Ask questions, "What's it for, and is it necessary?" until you feel that you have a level of informed consent that helps you feel safe.

Hire a birth worker, Doula or midwife to help advocate your needs.

---

* Sacred Mother: A video embracing sensual form- ripe with creation amidst an electrical storm. https://bit.ly/sacredmothervideo

Double-check hospital protocols to see if they are allowed into the birthing space.

Slow down, unplug and tap into your sensual nature as a ripening woman, integrate your inner Maiden and begin to activate the Birth Field.

Explore the erotic energy of being ripe with creation. Remember the same energy that got your baby in there, will help get your baby out.

Allow yourself to soften and surrender to your body's wisdom and start to encourage the flow of oxytocin.

Lineage

Pregnancy allows us to connect with the women in our bloodlines more intimately. It's as if you are suddenly granted access to a secret club you knew was there, but it now lands more viscerally for you as a lived experience. As you slowly emerge into your new identity as a mother, your perspective of ancestral stories will shift and a newfound compassion may arise in your heart and mind as if a veil is lifted and you can see with more depth and clarity. You may start to wonder what your grandmothers went through during their pregnancies and birth, how the zeitgeist affected their experiences of being initiated from *Maiden to Mother* and how that related to the way they reared their children- your ancestors. You may have to sit with and reconcile the fact that some of these women may have been children at the time or were impregnated nonconsensually. There may be scandal, brutality and trauma, just as there will be creativity, strength, and kindness. You will most likely discover a full spectrum of the human condition played out and begin to wonder what you've been imprinted with, what stories and beliefs were passed down the line that you still carry unconsciously, and what cycles you can now let go of and lay to rest.

When you look at your grandmothers as the matriarchs of your lineage, you will see what cycles they had to break, what pain they had to endure and what wisdom and strength they have passed on down the line for you to be the beautiful and unique woman you are today. If you can access your ancestral lineage and family tree, you may be able to conceptualise what life was like for these women based on written or oral history and legacy.

It's incredibly mind-blowing to scale out to 10 generations and realise that it means 1,024 people existed for you to be here today, 512 of those were mothers. Only 10 are your direct matrilineal mothers, meaning you are directly connected from mother to daughter. From womb, to womb, to womb.

KNOWING what we know now about limbic imprinting, how you existed as an egg inside your mother's foetus as she resided inside your grandmother's womb- your womb line directly links you 3 generations at a time, back in time. If you can wrap your head around that, you can understand the power of being a cycle breaker of ancestral wounds. Your birthright is your power to liberate your lineage and begin to acknowledge the strength, wisdom, creativity and resilience that flows through your veins.

And now, it's your turn to take your seat as a living ancestor and matriarch of your own lineage. What a blessing it is for you to be here and honour all the women who have walked before you!

Womb Grid

When you become pregnant, you soften and surrender to the fullness of the feminine. It is not uncommon to feel alone on this journey, and you may feel isolated as it feels like everything is happening to you and within you. You are essentially alone on this experience with your child. Growing and nurturing a new life is an intense journey that commands energy. Pregnancy takes nutrients from your body and bones. It can also be quite taxing energetically as you are extra sensitive and receptive, especially during the ripening stages of pregnancy, as you begin to feel like you are walking between worlds acting as a sacred bridge.

Every woman is spiritually connected from womb to womb, creating a worldwide energetic womb web. If you allow yourself to expand on this you can start to imagine every single woman who is pregnant at the same time as a special demographic of the global population Each growing child, nestled in the fertile womb of a Mother is a beautiful spark of radiant light and these invisible threads of connection which span the entire globe, activate what I call the *Mamamatrix,* or more simply- *Womb Grid.*

As a mother enters the birthing field, she can access the collective wisdom of this *Womb Grid,* which allows her to connect with a global sisterhood of birthing mothers who are labouring simultaneously. The power and majick of this is that a birthing mother is never alone. You are connected to something bigger through the vast, expansive shamanic dimensions of pregnancy and birth.

The *Womb Grid* is like an invisible mycelial network that exists in all moments and spans all timelines across all dimensions. It supports the grand tapestry and sacred web of life, *The Great Mystery.* The grid draws upon the collective sacred feminine energy. It helps to stabilise the birth field, which allows women to access the interdimensional portals they must traverse, acting as the sacred bridge between worlds to bring the baby through, Earthside.

IN THE SHAMANIC dimensions of Birth, time as we know it ceases to exist. In this space, a birthing mother enters the realms of the timeless and can access the wisdom and strength of all past, present and future birthing mothers. I call this the *Primal Wild,* which is only accessible during birth. In this place, you can also tap into unprecedented energy and use it to birth new dreaming and powerful visions alongside your baby, awakening powerful new majick to share with the world. As you birth your baby, you birth new worlds and visions for the future.

The first time I did this was during my first free birth at home. I was so silent and focused in this shamanic dimension that I received a powerful vision of my purpose work beyond the legacy of being a loving, present mother. At that moment, I touched upon the threads of my lineage, connecting with all of my grandmothers, breathing their strength and wisdom into my being as I breathed my daughter through quietly, gently and gracefully.

. . .

I AM a strong believer in the notion that we have the power to change the world in one generation. Imagine a world where ripe, heavily pregnant women were consciously dreaming a shared vision of a beautiful and peaceful new world and birthing it together!

Activating the Womb Grid Meditation

This meditation is designed to connect you with the ancient lineage of women in your bloodline, honour the sacred journey of pregnancy and activate the *Womb Grid*. By tapping into this collective wisdom and strength, you will feel supported, empowered and deeply connected to the primal wildness and majick of birthing.

To begin, find a quiet, comfortable space where you will not be disturbed. You may wish to light a candle, play soft music, or have objects that symbolise femininity and motherhood around you.

Sit or lay down comfortably, with your hands resting on your blossoming belly. If you're heavily pregnant, lay on your left side and use pillows to support your bump. Close your eyes and take a few deep breaths, inhaling through your nose and exhaling through your mouth. With each breath relax deeply, softening your shoulders and jaw. Allow yourself to breathe with a long rhythmic breath that feels good.

Now visualise a warm, golden light forming at the base of your spine. As you inhale, allow this light to travel up through your body, filling you with warmth and peace. As the light reaches your heart, imagine it expanding outward, creating a cocoon of golden light around you and your baby. In this cocoon, invite the presence of your female ancestors, your mother, grandmothers, and all the women who came before them. Feel their loving, supportive energy surrounding you.

Reflect on the journeys these women have undertaken, the strength they have shown and the wisdom they have passed down. Acknowledge their struggles, their triumphs, and the lessons they have imparted.

Now, imagine your womb as a radiant, glowing centre of light. This light begins to extend outward, connecting with the wombs of all pregnant women around the world. Visualise a vast, intricate web of light, the *Womb Grid*, a powerful network of shared energy, wisdom, and support. Feel the strength and love flowing through this grid. Know that you are not alone on this journey; you are connected to a global sisterhood of mothers.

As you breathe in, draw in the collective energy and wisdom of the *Womb Grid*. As you breathe out, send your love, wisdom and strength back into the grid.

When you feel connected to the grid begin to breathe more deeply and rhythmically. In your mind's eye, imagine yourself standing at the edge of a great, ancient forest, a place that represents the *Primal Wild*, the timeless realm of birthing mothers.

Step into this forest, feeling the earth beneath your feet and the vibrant energy of life around you. Here, time ceases to exist. You are surrounded by the spirits of past, present and future birthing mothers, all of whom lend you their strength and guidance. Allow yourself to be fully present in this space, open to receiving any messages, visions, or insights that may come to you.

As you stand in the *Primal Wild,* envision the birth of your baby as a powerful, transformative event. See yourself bringing new life and new dreams into the world. Imagine the world you wish to create for your child, a world filled with peace, love, and beauty. See other pregnant women around the world sharing this vision, collectively dreaming a new reality. Feel the energy of this shared vision flowing through you, empowering you to bring forth not just a new life, but a new way of being.

Allow yourself to open to the opportunities that align with your highest and most aligned potential in this lifetime. Imagine the support, resources and relationships that will be needed to help birth this and breathe awareness, vitality and life into this potential. Stay here for as long as it feels good.

Gradually bring your awareness back to the golden cocoon of light surrounding you and your baby. Take a few deep breaths, grounding yourself back in your physical body. When you are ready, open your eyes, carrying with you the wisdom, strength, and support of your ancestors, the *Womb Grid*, and the *Primal Wild*.

. . .

TAKE a moment to honour yourself and the incredible journey you are on. Know that you are a living ancestor, a matriarch in your own right, connected to a vast lineage of powerful women through the *Womb Grid*. You may forget at times, but you are never truly alone; you are part of a global sisterhood of sensually alive, majickal and powerful wise women.

I hope this meditation* reminds you of your strength and capacity to create and nurture new worlds. As with any journey work, make sure you take time to regulate and integrate, especially if you experience emotional responses. Give yourself some time to rest and resplenish.

---

* *I've created a recording of this guided journey, which is available for free on my website here: www.donnaraymond.com.au/WombGridMeditation*

8

NOURISHING THE JOURNEY
EMBRACING WHOLE BODY NUTRITION

"Mothers and babies form an inseparable biological and social unit; the health and nutrition of one group cannot be divorced from the health and nutrition of the other."
-*World Health Organization*

Every woman's nutritional needs during pregnancy and postpartum are unique and may vary based on age, weight, pre-existing health conditions, activity level and dietary preferences. While prenatal supplements can be beneficial for filling nutrient gaps, they should not replace a healthy diet based on whole, nutrient-dense foods. Whole foods provide a wide array of vitamins, minerals, antioxidants and other phytonutrients that are essential for supporting pregnancy and fetal development. Emphasising a diet rich in fruits, vegetables, whole grains, lean proteins and healthy fats can provide the necessary nutrients for a healthy pregnancy and postpartum recovery.

Staying hydrated is crucial as mineral-rich water plays a vital role in supporting various bodily functions, including digestion, circulation, and nutrient transport. Pregnant women should aim to drink plenty of water throughout the day and pay attention to signs of dehydration, such as dark urine or thirst. Herbal teas, coconut water, and fresh fruits can also contribute to hydration while providing additional nutrients.

OPTIMAL NUTRITION IS crucial during pregnancy to support the health and development of both the mother and the baby. Here are 30 nutrient-dense foods that can be beneficial during pregnancy:

- **Leafy Greens:** Rich in folate, iron, calcium, and vitamins A, C, and K. (e.g. Spinach, kale, Swiss chard etc.)
- **Legumes:** Excellent sources of protein, fibre, iron, folate, and zinc. (e.g. Lentils, chickpeas, black beans)
- **Avocado:** High in healthy fats, fibre, folate, potassium, and vitamins C, E, and K.
- **Sweet Potatoes:** Packed with beta-carotene, fibre, vitamin C, potassium, and B vitamins.
- **Salmon** (wild-caught): Rich in omega-3 fatty acids, protein, vitamin D, and B vitamins.
- **Eggs:** Excellent source of protein, choline, and essential vitamins and minerals. (Farm fresh or free-range is best)
- **Greek Yogurt:** High in protein, calcium, probiotics, and B vitamins.
- **Berries:** Loaded with antioxidants, fibre, and vitamins C and K. (e.g. Blueberries, strawberries, raspberries)
- **Nuts and Seeds:** Provide healthy fats, protein, fibre, vitamins, and minerals. (e.g. Almonds, walnuts, chia seeds)
- **Quinoa:** Complete protein source, rich in fibre, iron, magnesium, and folate.
- **Broccoli:** Packed with fibre, folate, calcium, vitamin C, and other antioxidants.
- **Lean Beef:** Excellent source of high-quality protein, iron, zinc, and B vitamins. (source local grass-fed beef)
- **Dairy:** Rich in calcium, protein, vitamin D, and probiotics. (e.g., milk, cheese, yogurt)

- **Oranges:** High in vitamin C, fibre, and antioxidants.
- **Bell Peppers:** Excellent source of vitamin C, vitamin A, and antioxidants.
- **Tomatoes:** Rich in vitamin C, potassium, and lycopene.
- **Pumpkin Seeds:** Provide protein, healthy fats, iron, zinc, magnesium, and fibre.
- **Edamame:** High in protein, fibre, folate, and iron.
- **Dark Chocolate:** Contains antioxidants, iron, and magnesium, and may help improve mood. (in moderation)
- **Seaweed** (e.g., nori, kelp): Rich in iodine, calcium, iron, and other minerals.
- **Oats:** Good source of fibre, protein, iron, and B vitamins.
- **Chia Seeds:** Provide omega-3 fatty acids, fibre, protein, and calcium.
- **Whole Grain Bread and Pasta:** Rich in fibre, B vitamins, and minerals.
- **Mangoes:** High in vitamin C, vitamin A, fibre, and antioxidants.
- **Bananas:** Good source of potassium, vitamin C, vitamin B6, and fibre.
- **Cottage Cheese:** High in protein, calcium, and B vitamins.
- **Kiwi:** Rich in vitamin C, vitamin K, potassium, and fibre.
- **Brussels Sprouts:** Packed with fibre, vitamin C, vitamin K, and antioxidants.
- **Peanut Butter:** Provides protein, healthy fats, vitamin E, and magnesium.

Unraveling the Mystery of Cravings:

PREGNANCY CRAVINGS CAN MANIFEST in a variety of ways, ranging from the mundane to the bizarre, and can strike at any time of day or night. While some cravings may be purely driven by taste preferences or cultural influences, others may be the body signalling specific nutritional deficiencies. Understanding the underlying reasons behind cravings can provide valuable insights into how to address them effectively while supporting maternal and foetal health. Certain cravings during pregnancy have been linked to common nutritional deficiencies, highlighting the importance of addressing these deficiencies through dietary choices or supplementation.

FOR EXAMPLE:

- **Craving for Ice:** An intense craving for ice, known as *pagophagia*, may indicate Iron Deficiency Anemia. Iron-rich foods such as lean meats, dark leafy greens and legumes can help address this deficiency. Adding Vitamin C to your diet creates an acid environment that will help increase iron absorption by 30%, whereas dairy will inhibit it. I experienced this during one of my pregnancies and a friend told me it was a sign of anemia, which I had later confirmed with a blood test.
- **Desire for Sour Foods:** Cravings for sour foods like citrus fruits or pickles may indicate a need for vitamin C, which is crucial in immune function and collagen synthesis. It also helps boost iron absorption. Keep this in mind if you're on an iron supplement.
- **Craving for Chocolate:** While chocolate cravings are common and may be driven by factors like mood enhancement, they may also signal a magnesium deficiency. Incorporating magnesium-rich foods such as nuts, seeds, whole grains and leafy greens can help meet this need. If you supplement, ensure the magnesium is bio-active and easily absorbed in the body.
- **Longing for Red Meat:** A strong desire for red meat may suggest a need for iron and protein, particularly common during the second and third trimesters of pregnancy. Including lean red meats, poultry, fish and plant-based iron sources like lentils and tofu can help address this deficiency.
- **Pica:** Refers to the craving for substances that offer little to no nutritional value and are often caused by an underlying

medical condition or deficiency. Most pregnancy pica revolves around the consumption of items such as ice, dirt, cardboard, chalk, etc.; however, less common items include glue, hair, toothpaste, rubber and toilet paper. It's important to seek medical advice if you suspect pica and try to substitute it with texturally similar food-based alternatives. For example, ground-up biscuits mixed with cacao could be a similar sensory experience to eating dirt.

It's important to listen to your body's cravings and preferences while ensuring you meet your nutritional needs with a varied and balanced diet during pregnancy.

Bone Broth

Bone broth is a sacred food that provides essential nutrients for pregnant women and supports postpartum recovery. It offers several nutritional benefits due to its rich nutrient profile and easy digestibility. Bone broth has a rich cultural and historical significance in many societies where it has been valued as a nourishing and healing food for pregnant women and new mothers. Its use during pregnancy and postpartum reflects the belief in its ability to provide essential nutrients, support warmth in recovery and promote overall well-being during these critical life stages.

In Chinese culture, it is often recommended to pregnant women and new mothers as a nourishing and fortifying food. Bone broth is considered to have *'qi'* (life energy) and blood-nourishing properties, which are important for supporting maternal health, replenishing lost nutrients, and promoting lactation.

In Ayurvedic tradition, a watery broth known as *'yusha'* is considered a deeply nourishing food for pregnancy and postpartum. It is believed to support digestive health, strengthen the immune system and provide vital nutrients for both mother and baby. Ayurvedic practitioners may recommend specific herbs and spices to add to the broth to enhance its therapeutic properties, depending on the individual's constitution and needs.

In traditional European folk medicine, broth made from simmering bones and vegetables is often recommended during pregnancy and postpartum to promote recovery, boost energy levels and support overall health. It is believed to be particularly beneficial for replenishing lost nutrients and aiding in the healing process after childbirth.

In many Native American cultures, bone broth has been a staple food for generations, valued for its nourishing and healing properties. It is often made from wild game such as deer or bison and herbs and roots may be added for additional flavour and medicinal benefits.

Broth can be consumed as a comforting and nourishing drink or as a base for soups, stews, sauces and other recipes. Bone Broth, in particular, has a strong beneficial nutrient profile that varies depending on the added ingredients but, for the most part, includes the following:

- **Rich in Nutrients:** Bone broth is made by simmering animal bones (such as chicken, beef, or fish) with water and aromatic vegetables for an extended period, which extracts valuable nutrients such as collagen, gelatin, vitamins, and minerals from the bones. These nutrients include calcium, magnesium, phosphorus, and potassium, essential for bone health, muscle function, and overall vitality during pregnancy and postpartum.
- **Supports Connective Tissue Health:** Collagen and gelatin, two prominent components of bone broth, are beneficial for supporting the health of connective tissues, including skin, joints, and ligaments. During pregnancy, when the body undergoes significant changes and increased strain on the musculoskeletal system, consuming collagen-rich foods like bone broth may help support joint health and reduce discomfort.
- **Gut Healing and Digestive Support:** The gelatin in bone broth has a soothing effect on the digestive tract and may help repair and strengthen the gut lining. This can be particularly beneficial during pregnancy and postpartum, as digestive issues such as constipation, bloating, reflux and heartburn are common due to hormonal changes and increased pressure on the digestive organs.

- **Hydration and Nourishment:** Bone broth is hydrating and easy to digest, making it a convenient way to stay hydrated and nourished, especially during the postpartum period when hydration and nutrient intake are crucial for recovery and breastfeeding support.
- **Boosts Immune Function:** The amino acids and minerals found in bone broth, such as glycine and zinc, support immune function and may help strengthen the body's defences against infections and illnesses. This can be particularly important during pregnancy and postpartum when the immune system may be more vulnerable.

Simple Bone Broth Recipe

Ingredients:

- 1-2kg beef, chicken, or fish bones (organic is ideal)
- 2 carrots, washed and chopped (do not peel)
- 2 celery stalks, chopped
- 1 onion, quartered
- 4 cloves of garlic, smashed
- 2 bay leaves
- Water
- Optional: apple cider vinegar (to help extract minerals from the bones)

Instructions:

1. Place the bones in a large stockpot or slow cooker.
2. Add chopped vegetables, garlic, bay leaves, and a splash of apple cider vinegar
3. Cover the bones and vegetables with water, ensuring they are fully submerged.
4. Bring the water to a boil, then reduce the heat to low and simmer, covered, for at least 8 hours (up to 24 hours for

maximum flavour and nutrient extraction). Alternatively, cook in a slow cooker on low for 12-24 hours.
5. Skim off any foam or impurities that rise to the surface during cooking.
6. Once the broth is done cooking, strain it through a fine-mesh sieve or cheesecloth to remove the solids.
7. Allow the broth to cool, then store it in glass jars or containers in the refrigerator for up to one week or freeze for longer storage.

Plant Allies

Turning to the power of plant medicine to support you through pregnancy, birth and motherhood is a beautiful way to feel connected to the inherent wisdom of the natural world. Generally speaking, most herbal remedies are safe to use. However, everybody is different and some herbal remedies are incredibly potent, so working closely with a herbalist, traditional Chinese, or functional medicine practitioner will help you explore remedies and the correct dosage for your body. Here is a list of some of my favourite simple plant medicines to assist you on your journey.

- **Alfalfa leaf:** Supports lactation and is a safe herb to take while pregnant. Alfalfa is rich in chlorophyll and vitamin K, a nutrient necessary for blood clotting. In the last trimester of pregnancy, alfalfa can decrease postpartum bleeding or the chance of hemorrhaging. You can purchase Alfalfa from most health food shops. Brew as a loose-leaf tea and eat the sprouts in salads or on their own.
- **Chamomile:** Helps control pain during labour by relieving tension, is also fantastic for helping reduce stress, and is great for sleepy time tea.
- **Fennel Seed:** Perhaps the most commonly used herb to support lactation. Fennel is a digestive herb that can help to relieve heartburn, gas, colic, and an upset tummy. You can

also put crushed seeds in hot water and use them as a warm compress for swollen and tender breasts from nursing.
- **Fenugreek seed:** Another popular herb for boosting lactation supply! *Caution- Do not use it during pregnancy because it's a uterine stimulant.*
- **Nettle:** Fantastic herb to drink as a tea packed full of Iron and vitamins A and C. It helps to support anaemia and healthy adrenal function. I started drinking this at around 36 weeks in preparation. I continued through my breastfeeding journey with Alfalfa to aid in a healthy milk supply and vitamin K because I did not vaccinate my children.
- **Moringa Leaf:** Rich in vitamins A, C, and E, calcium, and antioxidants. It helps to increase iron levels, reduces malnutrition and micronutrient deficiencies, and provides warmth to the body. It may cause uterine contractions, so use it during your postpartum recovery.
- **Raspberry Leaf:** Is one of the best uterine tonic herbs to prepare uterine muscles for efficient labour. Seriously, this stuff is amazing! It also helps to slow bleeding and expel the placenta. Have the tea on hand or make raspberry tea ice cubes to suck on during labour. I started drinking the tea around 36 weeks, and my 2nd and 3rd active labours were 90 minutes, and my 4th was 60 minutes. The leaves contain calcium, magnesium, and iron and can relieve diarrhoea and nausea. This is one of the best herbs for women. A great all-rounder as a tea or tincture!
- **Sweet Leaf:** Also known as Katuk or tropical asparagus, it is a valuable survival food great for blood building and cell rejuvenation and is beneficial to circulation, gut flora and bowel health. 25 grams daily for 14 days of Sweet Leaf mixed with lemon juice can help anemic mothers boost their hemoglobin levels. It can help increase milk production and is high in protein and fibre, which makes it a great food for vegetarians. It contains Iron, Magnesium, Potassium, Calcium and vitamins A, B, and C. Eat fresh, toss them in a salad, fry them up or add to cooked dishes.

Herbal Tinctures

- **Blue/Black Cohosh:** Two herbs that work synergistically to bring on labour (but do not use before the 39th week of pregnancy). They can make contractions more efficient during long, stalled labour and help the uterus clamp down after birth. I tried a natural induction at 40+6 weeks, but alas, my secondborn was quite stubborn, and it didn't work as she wasn't quite ready to come.
- **Motherwort:** This herb is bitter. I used it in tincture form and think of it as medicine. It is great for anxiety or when you're having a day of overwhelm, and you feel like you want to run away. A few drops under the tongue, and within a few minutes, balance and peace are restored. It helps to take the edge off. Phew!
- **Skullcap:** Helps to relax the nervous system- another great one for new mamas who are overthinking things and struggling with adapting to the changes a newborn brings or if you feel 'touched out' and overstimulated (it happens!)
- **Shepherd's Purse:** This is known to be the best herb to stop postpartum haemorrhaging quickly! It's a must-have for all birth workers.
- **Angelica Root:** Helps with circulation and is known to be a women's herb because of its ability to stimulate blood flow. Angelica can help relieve menstrual cramping by helping with warming, relaxing, decongesting and stimulating flow. It has been used as an afterbirth tonic to help expel the placenta and can also be used to regulate the menstrual cycle and bring on delayed menses

Essential Oils

- **Clary Sage:** should only be used in labour or to induce labour. It is a powerful oil that helps support and relieve tension during the powerful labour surges. I diffused in my birth suite, though you can also apply diluted and massage the belly during the transition phase- be mindful that it is a very strong-smelling aroma.

- **Frankincense**: Frankincense is a powerful all-rounder of the essential oil world. It has been used for centuries for its grounding and spiritually uplifting properties. Frankincense oil may help reduce stress, support emotional balance, and enhance spiritual connection during pregnancy. In labour, frankincense oil can be diffused or applied topically (diluted) to promote feelings of peace, strength and inner calm. It has powerful anti-inflammatory properties and can help connect you with your aligned vision for birth and beyond. Frankincense has been used in many cultures for its powerful spiritual energy and has become a revered resin for rituals and ceremonies. Diffuse in your Birth Space, anoint with 1 drop on your third eye, or use topically on the shoulders and legs to promote deep stillness and relaxation.
- **Jasmine**: Known as the king of the flowers, Jasmine helps to connect you to your sacred sexuality and the sacredness of birth. It can induce uterine contractions to help labour progress. Like Clary Sage, it is not recommended during your pregnancy. Jasmine can naturally strengthen contractions while providing natural pain relief and smells incredible! Purchase as a roller for easy topical application.
- **Lavender**: Its relaxing qualities can help keep you calm during the surges, and because it has powerful analgesic properties, it can help relieve tension in your aching muscles. It is great to diffuse or apply in a roller blend with frankincense for a powerful anti-inflammatory blend.
- **Melissa/Lemon Balm**: Helps to connect us to the Divine Feminine. She is deeply relaxing and grounded in her presence. Known as the oil of light, she can help connect us to our inner light and help guide the baby through clearly. It is great to diffuse in your birth space.
- **Rose**: Considered to be one of the highest vibrational plant medicines, rose oil is known as the oil of divine love and

can help you to surrender deeper into your love as a birthing mother, assisting you to open and expand the pelvis, helping the baby to pass through. Rose can rejuvenate tired skin, soften ligaments, and cleanse the uterus. Rose is a beautiful gift and one of the most precious and sacred oils.
- **Copaiba:** Sourced from the bark of a few different species of Amazonian trees, Copaiba is known as the oil of revealing. It is particularly great for deep shadow work and revealing what is hidden. It has powerful pain-relieving qualities as it works directly with the Endocannabinoid System via the CB2 receptor sites. Use during labour to help ease tension from rising surges.
- **Roman Chamomile:** Roman chamomile is another gentle and calming essential oil that can be beneficial during pregnancy and birth. It is known for its anti-inflammatory and sedative properties, making it useful for relieving muscle tension, easing anxiety and promoting relaxation. Roman chamomile oil can be diffused or used in massage (diluted) to support emotional well-being and ease discomfort during labour.
- **Ylang Ylang:** Is renowned for its sweet, floral aroma and calming effects on the nervous system. During pregnancy, ylang-ylang oil may help alleviate anxiety, promote relaxation, and uplift the mood. In labour, ylang-ylang oil can be diffused or used in massage (diluted) to reduce tension, enhance relaxation and support emotional well-being.

Whole Body Nutrition

Pregnancy is a time of heightened awareness of the body's innate wisdom and needs. Listening to the subtle cues and signals your body sends you is essential as you nourish yourself and your growing baby. This means tuning into hunger and fullness cues, cravings and preferences and honouring them with whole, nutrient-dense foods supporting maternal and fetal health. You can foster a deeper connection to your body and the life growing within by approaching nutrition with curiosity, mindfulness and self-compassion.

Whole-body nutrition encompasses more than just the physical aspects of nourishment; it encompasses the emotional, spiritual and relational dimensions of your experience with food as medicine. During pregnancy and postpartum, you can nourish yourself on all levels, nurturing your body, mind and Spirit with foods that promote vitality, balance and well-being. This may also involve incorporating mindfulness practices such as meditation, gratitude, or breathwork into your daily routines and seeking support from loved ones, healthcare providers and community resources to navigate the ups and downs of this transformative journey.

Preparing and consuming food during pregnancy and postpartum can be a sacred ritual imbued with intention, gratitude and mindfulness. Whether sourcing fresh seasonal ingredients, engaging in mindful cooking practices, singing blessings over your cooking, growing your own food and tending to it with love or simply savouring each bite with presence and awareness. Meal preparation becomes an opportunity to nourish your body, mind and soul. Taking the time to slow down, breathe and connect with the natural world can enhance your appreciation for food's nourishing, life-giving power and deepen your connection to the experience of pregnancy and motherhood.

EXTENDING on from that is being mindful of the sensory input you consume daily and being conscious of how it can alter the way you think and feel. During pregnancy, you will be more sensitive to sensory information and considering you are constantly providing sensory information and imprinting on your newborn you need to be mindful of what you expose yourself to, what information you consume and how often. Fill your heart and mind with joyful and fun experiences and relationships that nourish your mind and heart and make you feel safe, creative, relaxed and inspired. Follow your bliss, still your mind and connect with your body. Limit the 'junk' and increase the Soul food intake.

Amid your *Maiden to Mother* journey, it is vital to create moments of stillness. A place to simply be and breathe. A sacred space where you feel safe to pause, reflect and become present with the subtle changes that are taking place. Walking barefoot in nature, eliminating distractions and the cacophony of stimuli the modern world bombards upon you, will help your nervous system regulate into a state of peace.

You must prioritise ways to recharge your Spirit from the massive task of pregnancy. Growing a human inside of you is no small feat, let alone raising a child in a kind, present and loving way.

Take time to connect with how sacred this transition is and relish in the miracle of life and your power as a mother.

9

BIRTH WARRIOR
OVERCOMING FEAR AND WORRY

"Birth takes a woman's deepest fears about herself and shows her that she is stronger than them."
– Unknown

Fear emerges instinctively when faced with unfamiliar or uncertain circumstances, activating your nervous system as a protective mechanism for survival. It often shrouds the sanctity of childbirth, obscuring its beauty and profound transformative power. Despite appearing and feeling real, fear lacks substance or tangible form; it is often irrational, conjured from the mind's worst-case scenarios or echo chambers of past negative experiences and inherited beliefs.

The initiatory power of birthing will bring you to your edges phenomenally. So much of the physiological process of birth as a lived experience is yet to be defined, as is your power as a woman; a mother who gives birth.

It takes strength to face your fears, to ask questions and to sit with the answers and the deep truths that call for your attention. It takes courage to look at all the negative and painful stories, to challenge and disrupt the modus operandi of the status quo and come to a place of acceptance for what is and is yet to be defined. The reality you truly face is your fear of death...the ultimate mystery.

To live life fully means to accept the ultimate truth, that death comes for us all eventually. It is a natural part of life, intrinsically linked to birth and a journey we all must face eventually. We so often forget the primal wisdom inherent in nature itself.

From Worrier to Warrior

The most challenging domain to master is the space between your ears; yet, in doing so, you unlock the door to extraordinary power. Fear possesses the psyche. It is a mind parasite that needs to be detoxed regularly, or it hijacks our creative power, binds us in its grip and renders us immobile. We shape our reality with our thoughts. Energy flows where attention goes.

The wisest path is to become a warrior, not a worrier. Investing your mental and emotional energy in what makes you feel powerless serves no purpose. You must take the lead, steering your life and your birth experience in the direction you desire, becoming more self-aware, enlightened and attuned to the deeper aspects of existence and your power as a birthing woman.

The energy of the Warrior embodies qualities of strength, courage and discipline, both in facing external challenges and confronting inner struggles. This archetype transcends mere physical combat, emphasising a journey of self-discovery and transformation.

Integrating aspects of the divine feminine, the *Birth Warrior* embodies compassion, intuition, and interconnectedness, fostering a harmonious balance between action and receptivity, strength and vulnerability. Ultimately, the warrior's path leads to inner peace, wisdom and alignment with a higher purpose. The *Birth Warrior* assesses risk and danger and prepares to make the necessary choices that lead to the desired outcome.

In the crucible of consciousness, you hold the key to your liberation, for within the vast expanse of the mind lies the power to birth your dreams into reality. Become a *Birth Warrior* and face your fears, feel your fears, but do not feed them. When you let go of fear and worry, you open the door to creativity and problem-solving.

This shift doesn't signify a lack of care or complacency with risks; rather, it reflects a deliberate choice to channel your energy into educating and empowering yourself with the wisdom and support necessary for the best possible journey. When fear serves as a motivator rather than a paralyser, it fosters mental fortitude, preparation and emotional resilience, bringing you closer to your creative power and what is truly meaningful.

Redefining Pain

In 2011, I came across a groundbreaking TEDx Talk called, *'Why Things Hurt'*[1] by clinical neuroscientist Lorimer Moseley. Professor Moseley hilariously delivers an entertaining and educational speech around the neurological fact that pain is not real. He states that,

> "Pain is an output of the brain designed to protect you… 100% Pain is a construct of the brain."

Pain is an illusion the brain produces and projects from sensory input to which we have assigned meaning. Aside from death, one of the biggest fears I hear pregnant women speak about is the physical pain of childbirth. The expected pain of the body stretching and opening for a few pounds of flesh to emerge.

Some women are so scared of this that they will elect to have a cesarean to avoid natural vaginal birth, not fully grasping that they are trading off this initiatory 'pain' for major abdominal surgery and post-partum recovery whilst caretaking a newborn. Everything is relative to our perceptions and beliefs. For the most part, our media sensationalises the dramatisation of birth through the performance of screaming chaotic contortions because, on a very primal level, it arouses and excites us. Drama sells.

As a young *Maiden*, I heard childbirth likened to pushing a pineapple out of your vagina and being ripped from the inside out. Many women joked about the crowning and that I had to wait to understand, like it was some kind of sinister secret. But when I got to that point myself, I wondered what all the fuss was about. Sure, it was an intense sensation, but I wouldn't say that it was painful! Maybe I was the weird one?

Pain to me was not knowing my wrist was broken for 2 days and driving a manual car, screaming whilst shifting gears, looking at my dangling wrist and thinking that perhaps I should get that checked out. HA!

I was raised in the mid 80's in a small Australian town, where you just 'sucked it up' and got on with it. Physical pain was never acknowledged as something debilitating. It was simply a sensation you felt and then got on with life. So when it came to the 'excruciating pain' of childbirth, I had the belief that it couldn't be that bad, could it?

Rationally, I wondered if childbirth was so unbearably painful, then why would women willingly choose to go back a second, third or fourth time? And why did my mum say she loved pregnancy and birth? For the most part, your experience of pain often comes down to the stories you tell yourself and the beliefs you program your mind with.

So much of empowered birthing is detoxing the mind of unhealthy narratives and distortions of natural, physiological birth. Birthing a baby is uncomfortable, all initiations are. You are meant to become so radically uncomfortable in your old identity that you transform into the new, through this initiatory power, into your own.

PAIN IS sensory information in the body. Using your breath, you can create space around the sensation, space for presence to receive the information encoded within the pain. Pain without presence is tension and contracts the body further.

> "Believe me: if you are told that some experience is going to hurt, it will hurt. Much of pain is in the mind, and when a woman absorbs the idea that the act of giving birth is excruciatingly painful – when she gets this information from her mother, her sisters, her married friends, and her physician – that woman has been mentally prepared to feel great agony."
>
> — Ina May Gaskin, Midwife and Author.

In childbirth, you need to see pain as an invitation to expand bigger than the sensation. Using your breath, you command your power to envelop the sensation with the depth of presence; the only way out is through and in this way, you meet your edges and remember your power. The journey of contraction and expansion calls you inwards. Motion is lotion, so moving with the sensations and surges lubricates the body from friction.

∼

Who's Knocking on Birth's Door?

Several years ago, I attended a workshop with Jane Hardwicke Collings about her *Autumn Woman Harvest Queen* work. We briefly touched upon the different rites of passage women move through in life and how the woman you were in the past will show up at birth's door. I have experienced this enough to receive the medicine of this concept as a lived reality.

When labour begins, you are activating the birth process and entering a spiritual doorway that allows you to bring your baby into the world. Different aspects of yourself from various stages of your life will manifest in this space. This is all part of the profound initiation of birth and the reclamation of the maternal role. The playful child, the rebellious teenager, the innocent young woman at her first menstruation and the sexually awakened woman; all of these aspects will be present at the threshold of birth. Additionally, the energetic imprints they carry and the stories and information you have gathered about womanhood during these significant life stages will also emerge.

The biggest imprints revolve around blood and sex. It is helpful to do the inner shadow work and identify and unpack these before they show up unconsciously at the altar of birth.

Some of the questions to ask revolve around the following themes:

- Information and messages you received about what it means to be a woman.
- How do you feel safe in your body and in the world?

- Your connection to pleasure and pain.
- The invisible burdens women carry.
- How do you experience support or lack thereof?
- How elder women and peers have connected with or rejected you.
- Your connection to your inner authority and power.
- Your connection to innocence and wonder.
- What was happening in your life around the time of your first bleed and the first time you engaged in sexual intimacy/intercourse.
- Stories and beliefs around menstruation and whether it has been an empowering, disempowering experience, a non-event or a burden.
- Your connection to your blood.
- Your thoughts and feelings around women being primary caretakers.
- Your relationship to mother figures in your life- and how they showed up at these rites of passage.
- Your beliefs and fears around death.
- Your ability to receive love and support and feel connected to the community.
- Your ability to trust other women.
- Anything to do with your connection to your womb shows up, especially losses.
- Intergenerational trauma connected to being an empowered woman, etc.

As you begin to identify these significant moments and their energetic patterns, you may notice a recurring theme. This is valuable insight. Pay attention to whether there is an expanding or contracting energy around these moments, as this will help you identify the areas that require healing and integration. With any shadow work, the process involves uncovering, experiencing, healing and integrating.

It is important to do this deep healing work before you are at the threshold of birth so that you can crossover feeling clear and anchored in your body, knowing that there is no space for those old stories to play out or be imprinted on your new baby. This perspective gives you courage as a cycle breaker to confront the patterns, beliefs and behaviours you've inherited while investing your energy in the necessary healing and integration so that you are not only a conscious mother but also a powerful matriarch.

Make no mistake, this is a big task. It may seem overwhelming to clear ancestral lines for some, but I want to assure you that you don't have to do it all by yourself. Do what you can in the best way. Never underestimate how small, consistent changes can lead to significant long-term effects.

So, How do you clear the way?

- Somatic practices- dance, movement, pulsing
- EFT- Emotional Freedom Technique
- EMDR- Eye Movement Desensitisation Reprocessing
- Shamanic Journey work and ceremony
- WombSong Emotional Alchemy Practice
- Breathwork + Nervous system regulation.
- Journalling and creative expression.

Having said that, sometimes we take simplicity for granted. You could have the biggest breakthroughs and spiritual insights from walking barefoot on country, connecting with nature and simply allowing yourself to create the necessary space to feel what needs to come through. With clear intent, you can focus on what you need to do without complicating the journey.

In my experience, all of this 'stuff' starts to come up around 7 months pregnant as the baby takes up more space inside the womb and it feels like an energetic purge to clear the way for birth. There is a divine wisdom present as your baby prepares the way with you. You are not alone on this journey.

When you begin to explore and examine parts of your life, especially those involving trauma, remember that you're not delving into the trauma itself or immersing in the story and lived experience of it. Instead, focus on the core emotional imprints so you can heal and integrate them.

It is important to understand that when you delve into 'story' you can reanimate the trauma because your brain cannot differentiate between the past as a memory or lived experience in the present. That's how powerful our brains are. So, If this is your path to walk, it is imperative to connect with your baby in the womb and talk to your child and speak to them from the place of maternal safety. What this looks like is reassuring the Spirit of your child that you are doing some deep healing work, and it has nothing to do with them or the world they will live in. I used to rub my belly and say:

> "This is not what's happening right now, sweetheart- Mama is just feeling and moving old energy through my body so I can be more present for you and clear the way for us to have a beautiful birth together."

As you make your way through this book, you might feel things viscerally. In these moments and life in general, place your hands on your womb, connect with your baby and provide reassurance as you have your sensory experiences.

Shadow Work

Carl Gustav Jung was a Swiss psychologist and visionary who first coined the concepts of the Conscious/Subconscious Mind and the Shadow Self. [2] In Jungian psychology, the Shadow represents the parts of ourselves, thoughts and feelings that we cast aside into the shadows of the psyche because we do not want to face them, in fact, we think it is easier to disown them, suppress them and to only focus on what we perceive as the 'positive' and more desirable qualities of Self. This strategy is often an act of self-preservation, especially after experiencing abuse and trauma on any scale, which is all relative and unique to each individual.

This coping strategy works for a while, except the trouble with this is that eventually, these shadow emotions will seep into your life via unhealthy subconscious behaviours, beliefs, patterns and eruptions of emotion. If not faced, acknowledged, integrated and healed, these stagnant energies can fester like an open wound left untreated, which leads to more intense mental, emotional and physical health challenges. Our bodies are encoded with such incredible wisdom and memory, not only from our own experiences but those passed down to us from our ancestral lineages. Unresolved emotions are a core component behind most suffering we experience.

OVER THE YEARS, as a mentor and facilitator of transformational healing and womb work, I discovered that the womb is an ideal storage place for these shadow energies, our own and our partners. As an energy centre, the womb is incredibly fertile, regardless of the physical ability to conceive and carry a child. The womb can and will harbour emotion. It's a generator, so we have to check in to see what stories we are storing inside our wombspace.

The narrative that plays out though, is that pregnant women are just simply hormonal and have the ability to swing between extreme and conflicting emotions. Yes, to some degree, the cocktail of hormones coursing through your body plays a part, though I notice the outbursts take place for the simple reason that our society does not allow the space for women to express their raw and untamed truth. During pregnancy, you are so sensitive and receptive to energy that the emotions you purge might be the ones you are most afraid to speak, or to share honestly, because they can often be unpleasant and disruptive. These emotions are often not spoken about and are usually suffered in silence… because you're meant to be happy that you're pregnant, right? You're lucky that you're fertile.

WHAT IF THE conception of the baby was not a result of love or ideal circumstances? What if the baby was conceived through abuse or manipulation? What if an unintended pregnancy has left you feeling overwhelmed and unprepared, regardless of whether it's your first or fifth child? These feelings are completely valid and can manifest as concerns about the stability and future of a relationship, feeling unsafe and unsupported, lack of trust in others, fear of change, anger, grief, confusion, lack of control, anxiety, low self-worth and more. So, how does this relate to pregnancy and birth?

Well, what I have taken note of, by being entrusted with women's intimate stories and my own experiences, is that during pregnancy, as the baby grows and takes up more space, the womb will naturally purge any unresolved emotions and tension that is stored there. This can happen throughout the pregnancy, though the pattern that seems consistent is that this natural purging is prevalent between the transition of the second and third trimesters, right up until birth if need be. I believe the process is to clear the channels to bring the baby through clearly. I also believe that our children help us reveal these shadow emotions so that we may heal and embody our truth in Sovereignty. Reveal to heal.

Any unresolved emotion will most likely show up at the birth door.

Integrating the Shadow

Pregnancy and birth can reveal many aspects of our shadow that may lay dormant. Entering into the ripening stages of pregnancy, it is imperative to heal unresolved trauma or wounds from the past, particularly in relation to our own mothers. It is also important to face our subconscious fears around being a mother, sexuality, relationships, body image, etc.

Below, you will find a series of journal prompts that will help you to create an unfiltered sub-conscious stream in response. This will help you to reveal anything that might be hidden and requires healing before you give birth. It is a necessary part of 'the *great work*' to clear out any energetic debris so that you can be free to focus on birthing your baby with grace and love

As with any shadow work, it is essential to create a psychologically safe space to do this work and because of the fact that you are ripe with creation, it is also important to establish a psychic boundary between you and the baby so that it is not being fed any unpleasant emotions as they arise for integrating and healing. The more you become aware of the Shadow, the less control it has in playing out subconscious programs and beliefs in the background, manifesting undesirable outcomes that do not serve your highest potential.

The whole point of this exercise is to bring light to the shadow so that you can do the work to move through any blocks and emotions. Do not be afraid of this; the reality is that you have complete power over and choice of what you want to feel and experience in your life. If the responses come easy, these programs and beliefs have most likely become ingrained in your psyche as a 'norm' or 'truth'. The reason you want to identify these thoughts and internal narratives, no matter how irrational they might be, is so that you can re-write the script and change your mindset to one that fosters love, connection and confidence in your abilities to become an incredible mother that as an empowered birthing experience.

THESE ARE JUST PROMPTS, you can use them to create your own questions. When journalling, continue writing until you feel a change in your body, that's how you'll know the work is done. When I Journal in this way, I call it 'mapping' as you are exploring your inner worlds and using language to understand the terrain of yourself more clearly.

Once you have created your map, review your responses with love and acceptance. Learn what you need to move forward, consider conversations you may need to have now and think about ways you might want to improve relationships or set strong boundaries for yourself and your baby. When negative self-talk arises, challenge those thoughts and turn them around. This is a guide to help you connect more deeply with yourself, release any tension, frustration, or trapped emotions and open up to feelings of peace and expansion.

RELATIONSHIP

- I choose to admit that I am actually... about my relationship
- I secretly fear that...
- I worry that my partner...
- I worry that becoming a mother will affect my relationship... (how, in what ways?)
- (Partners name) won't be able to fully support me because...

- This makes me feel…
- I need to let my partner know that…
- If I died, I'm worried that…
- I'm worried that my partner will (name the fear- even if it is irrational) when the baby is here.
- I'm scared he/she won't find me attractive because…
- I worry about the stability of my relationship because…
- Being a Single Mother would make me feel…
- I'm worried that I'm going to be the one who always…

Becoming a Mother

- I'm not going to be a good enough Mother because…
- I'm scared I'm going to… (name fear)
- I'm scared my baby will…
- My life is never going to be the same, and it makes me feel…
- I'm worried that I'm going to screw my child up because…
- If I'm really honest with myself, I feel… about motherhood

Body Image

- I'm worried about the changes my body is going through, and I feel… about it.
- I'm scared that my vagina (or any other body part)…
- My baby-body is…
- I'm unhappy with my body because…
- I secretly wish my body was…
- I am scared my body will be…
- I'm worried if I don't get my pre-baby body back…

Release the Root

One of the best ways to quickly transmute any undesirable energy is first to identify it and to call it by its true name. One of the fundamental principles of *majick* is that you command control over something by calling it by its true name. It is easy to sense the emotion on the surface layer, though the journey of excavating the roots can prove to be much more of an inner journey.

Journalling is a powerful practice. If done correctly, it can help to identify deep subconscious fears and blocks. This allows clear insight into your inner landscape, so you can choose what stays and what is released in a loving and healing way. Many healing modalities can assist you in tapping into any hidden fears and resistance you may have around birth and becoming a mother. Working with someone who makes you feel safe and supported is best practice. This is not the time to dabble!

Alternative therapies such as Breathwork, Craniosacral, Kinesiology, EFT, EMDR, Holographic Kinetics, Somatic Respiratory Integration, Holistic Massage and Pulsing can all help with releasing tension and emotion trapped in the body, preparing it for a clear and beautiful birthing experience.

In my practice of emotional alchemy, called WombSong, I teach women how to connect with their wombspace and release any negative or leftover energy through sound. Sound is a powerful tool for accessing emotions and shifting energy, and since I first experienced the WombSong practice, it has become a regular ritual for me to cleanse myself and build emotional resilience. This is especially important because of my work facilitating intense forms of transformative healing.

Protect Your Field

As a pregnant mother, you most likely attract many different types of people who feel like they can give you unsolicited advice. Depending on where you live, you will probably experience comments and remarks about your changing body or choices that are not warranted. You may also find that friends and family members project their fears, worries and anxieties onto you and that other mothers voluntarily share their often dramatic and traumatic birth stories with you without permission. For some reason, being around a pregnant woman triggers this unconscious behaviour. Most of the time, it's coming from a need to be helpful and caring.

When you are ripe with creation, you are inherently more sensitive and receptive to energies around you, so it is important that you are discerning as to who you surround yourself with, what advice you take on and absorb, and what type of environment you place yourself into. This is especially important if you are deciding to homebirth or freebirth because not everyone will understand or agree with your choices. It is wise to share your plans with people who will help to encourage and empower you on your journey.

As a Maiden, it is absolutely essential that you are mindful of what type of information you expose yourself to (including social media) and also set firm boundaries in the way people communicate and relate to you.

Boundaries and Priorities

Remember, this is great work; you must be vigilant with your energetic boundaries to protect the sacred energy surrounding your pregnancy and the birth of your baby.

Every morning, set the intention of who you choose to connect with, what you will and will not tolerate and what boundaries need to be set in place or communicated with others to protect your field.

This might be initially uncomfortable, especially if you're a people pleaser. You may need to say no or remove yourself from certain situations. It is totally ok for you to interrupt someone who is sharing unsolicited advice or fear-mongering. You do not need to wait for that pause in the conversation to be polite because, most of the time, it doesn't come. You have to seize the moment and you do not owe anyone an explanation. Think of it as practice, stepping into your authority.

People who respect you will respect your boundaries.

The reality is that this time of pregnancy is precious and may only happen a few more times in your life. When you fully honour and respect your role as a Mother, it makes it easier to be the conscious custodian of this field and the sensory information your baby will be exposed to.

Before you go to bed, check in with the baby and have a moment to decompress and reflect upon the day. This will allow you to process any residual emotional energy, stress, doubts or tension you've picked up so you can consciously release it.

Crystals

Many people use crystals to harness their unique energies, which are thought to promote healing and balance in the body and mind. Try to source your crystals as ethically as possible and if you are fossicking, make sure you connect with the land and ask permission to take them. Always giving something back in return. An easy way to use crystals is to keep them inside your bra, wear them as jewellery or place them upon your altar in your sacred space. It's important to cleanse your crystals before you use them for the first time or if you're processing heavy emotions. There are several ways to do this, though I like to take my crystals down to the creek and let the freshwater flow over them for a few minutes. You can charge them in a bowl of water under the full moon and make 'moon water' and you can then use this water in a ritual or mix it with essential oil as a majickal spritz. Some spritz bottles are wide enough to fit crystal chips inside.

Here are several crystals known to help release fear and anxiety, especially related to pregnancy and childbirth:

- **Amethyst:** Known for its calming and protective energy, amethyst helps reduce anxiety and stress, promoting a sense of peace and stability. In addition to its calming properties, amethyst can help clear negative thoughts and emotions, promoting mental clarity and spiritual upliftment.
- **Aquamarine:** Associated with soothing and calming energies, aquamarine can help reduce stress and fear, promoting a peaceful state of mind.

- **Black Tourmaline:** This protective stone is thought to absorb negative energy and provide grounding, helping to alleviate fear and anxiety. Renowned for its protective qualities, black tourmaline is excellent at absorbing and transmuting negative energy, grounding and protecting the user from harm.
- **Citrine:** Often called the "stone of abundance," helps to dispel negative energy and bring in positive, prosperous vibes. It's great for transforming negative thoughts into positive ones.
- **Fluorite:** Known for its cleansing properties, fluorite helps to remove negative energies and balance the aura, making it useful for mental clarity and decision-making.
- **Hematite:** This grounding stone helps to absorb negative energy and calm in times of stress or worry. It also promotes a sense of stability and balance.
- **Lepidolite:** Known for its mood-stabilising properties, lepidolite can help reduce anxiety and promote a sense of calm and tranquillity.
- **Moonstone:** This crystal is associated with feminine energy and is believed to support fertility, pregnancy and childbirth while also easing stress and anxiety.
- **Obsidian:** A powerful protective stone, obsidian helps to shield against negativity and emotional blockages, promoting a clear and focused mind.
- **Rose Quartz:** Often called the "stone of love," rose quartz encourages self-love, emotional healing and a sense of calm, making it especially helpful during pregnancy and childbirth.
- **Selenite:** Known for its high vibrational energy, selenite can cleanse and purify negative energies from a space or person, creating a peaceful environment. Consider having a selenite lamp in your birth space.
- **Smoky Quartz:** This crystal is effective at neutralising negative vibrations and detoxifying energetic fields, making it great for cleansing spaces and personal energy.

Amulets and Talismans

FROM A MAJICKAL PERSPECTIVE, working with amulets and talismans is a powerful way to release what is not resonant and to anchor new beliefs and mindset practices. Sometimes, you need ways to reality hack, to stay focused on the adventures you choose repeatedly. Amulets and talismans were historically used to express the desire to become a Mother and to protect from childbirth risks.

From Antiquity to Byzantium, amulets resembling a uterus were used on a small part of the body to aid pregnancy and childbirth and to protect against the evil eye. These amulets were believed to prevent demons from harming and stealing women and children. Magical texts were also used for these purposes. Women's use of magic and amulets dates back to the 5th century BC.

Aetites, known as Eagle Stones, were worn as magical amulets across Northern Europe. They were believed to be carried by eagles to their nests to help in laying eggs and were said to prevent spontaneous abortion and premature labour in women. This magical stone is a type of geode where some of the crystalline structure has come loose. The folklore around this tells us that many believed the stone could give birth to other stones and so they were also known commonly as rattling stones, where the stone within a stone represented a child in the womb. According to Pedanius Dioscorides, the aetite, "should be fastened to the left arm to protect the fetus and at the time of birth should be removed to the hip area to ease birth."

A Holey Stone (Hagstone), hung over the bed where birth occurs, was believed to make delivery smoother and less painful. The hagstone is a natural stone with a hole through it, believed to have protective properties and to ward off negative energies and spirits during childbirth.

IN ADDITION TO PHYSICAL AMULETS, magical inscriptions and protection spells were used. A circle with magical inscriptions might be drawn around the bed to create a protective barrier. One notable example is the protection letter from Lilith in Jewish tradition. Lilith, often considered a demoness, was believed to pose a threat to women and infants. To protect against her, a letter of protection would be written and placed near the birthing woman, invoking divine guardians to ward off Lilith and other malevolent spirits.

These practices highlight the deep-seated belief in the power of symbols, stones and written words to influence and protect the birthing process. Women can draw on a rich history of protective and empowering rituals by incorporating these ancient traditions into modern birthing practices.

Worry Dolls

Worry dolls are small, handcrafted figures traditionally made from wood, wire and colourful textiles. These dolls are about 5cm tall, easily fit in the palm of your hand and are used to express and release fear, worry and anxiety symbolically. According to Guatemalan legends, worry dolls were placed under the pillow at night and by morning, the dolls would have alchemised the worry into wisdom and knowledge on how to overcome and eliminate it. East Slavic women made dolls during pregnancy in which they would put all their worry, fear, insecurity and unwanted energy of others. No one was allowed to see this doll, and it was discarded after the birth of her baby. The expectant mother would also make a doll for her child before birth, which would then be placed under the father's pillow to imbue it with protective energy.

10

THE POWER OF CEREMONY
WEAVING MEANING AND PURPOSE

"A ritual is the enactment of a myth.
And, by participating in the ritual, you are participating in the myth.
And since myth is a projection of the depth wisdom of the psyche, by participating in a ritual, participating in the myth, you are being, as it were, put in accord with that wisdom, which is the wisdom that is inherent within you anyhow. Your consciousness is being reminded of the wisdom of your own life."
–Joseph Campbell

In the intricate tapestry of life, ceremony plays a vital role in integrating *rites of passage,* profoundly impacting the collective human psyche, the health and well-being of communities and the maturation and spiritual evolution of the soul during times of transition. Ceremonies bridge the gap between the seen and unseen worlds, weaving the threads of individual stories with the collective mythos and infusing the mundane with majick.

Sacred ceremony offers an opportunity to step out of the ordinary everyday world and enter into a timeless realm, a sacred space where the natural seasons and cycles of life are honoured, where intentional thought is met with purposeful action and the ordinary becomes extraordinary.

Moments such as birth, coming of age, marriage and death are met with intention and create a world imbued with meaning, purpose, and connection, fostering the health and well-being of all beings.

In today's technocratic world of rapid change, the revival of the ceremonial arts is not only an act of rebellion from disconnection and distraction but a reclamation of human connection, depth and meaning. Sacred ceremonies and rituals create a space for individuals to step away from the frenetic and often frantic pace of modern life and reconnect with their inner selves, communities and of course, the natural world. They are safe containers for introspection, psychological processing and emotional regulation.

Through the engagement of intentional practice, individuals can unravel the hidden narratives woven within their psyche, making sense of the stories and patterns animated in the body through memory.

Rituals can awaken the inherent wisdom and power of the Spirit while facilitating the integration and closure of past events, the acceptance of a newfound identity and the embodiment of the wisdom gained from these lived experiences. For new mothers, ritual offers a framework for navigating the challenges and joys of motherhood, providing a sense of structure, meaning, and continuity amid constant change.

I've been a ceremonialist for nearly 20 years, guiding women through the seasons and cycles of life, death and rebirth. I have witnessed the profound impact of Sacred ceremonies and rituals on the human psyche. It is as though they activate a deep remembering within, a reminder to take your place within the grand tapestry of life, a call to create a life rich with meaning and purpose. A call to come home.

Blessingway

The *Blessingway* ceremony, originating from the Navajo people of the southwestern United States of America, holds deep cultural and spiritual significance as a sacred ritual to promote harmony, balance and well-being to bless the one that is to be 'sung over'.

Traditional Blessingway ceremonies, known as *Hózhójí*, are conducted by skilled Navajo singers or *Hataałii* (medicine people) and involve rituals, prayers and blessings aimed at honouring the sacredness of life, nature and the interconnectedness of all beings. Key elements include traditional songs and prayers, symbolic rituals of purification, the blessing of the mother's body, the sharing of wisdom from community members and the supportive presence of family and friends.

In Navajo culture, the Blessingway ceremony is deeply rooted in spirituality and cosmology, whereby symbolic and culturally significant rituals, such as smudging with sacred ceremonial herbs and anointing with oils, cleanse and purify the mother's body, preparing her for the journey of childbirth and motherhood.

While the Blessingway ceremony originates from Navajo culture, variations of this ritual have been embraced by people from diverse cultural backgrounds to honour and celebrate the journey of pregnancy and childbirth.

It is important to respect ancient cultural practices and not perform these customs without authority or permission. This is why I do not use the term Blessingway for any ceremonies and instead use the term Mother Blessing. When individuals or communities outside of Navajo culture appropriate the term 'Blessingway' to describe similar ceremonies or rituals, it can be deeply disrespectful and harmful. This appropriation can strip the ceremony of its cultural and spiritual context, trivialise its cultural and historical significance and contribute to the erasure or distortion of Navajo culture.

By promoting cultural understanding, respect, and reciprocity, we can foster meaningful cross-cultural exchange through appreciation while avoiding the harm of cultural appropriation.

Modern Mother Blessing Ceremony

You're probably familiar with the tradition of having a baby shower, right? It's an event where the expectant mother is showered with gifts in celebration and anticipation of the new arrival. Most of the time, baby showers are void of deep meaning and can be quite expensive.

A Mother Blessing, however, is something different altogether and aims to weave a web of support around the expectant Mother, with the sole focus being on nourishing her and offering blessings and prayers to her as she embarks on her sacred rite of passage.

With the focus on her, the expectant Mother will feel seen, heard, honoured and valued. I have had the pleasure of facilitating many Mother Blessing ceremonies and have drawn upon the wisdom of many different cultural traditions, each time honouring the sacred lineage with respect. Below, I will list a few potent and beautiful rituals you can use to create your ceremony or share with someone you trust so that they can create and facilitate it for you.

Sacred Bead Ritual

Origins in African/Native American traditions. You must share where these ceremonies come from. Sitting in a circle, the expectant mother will hold a long red string. She will then pass it to the woman sitting next to her. Ideally, the Mother's mother is the last person to place the bead. Each sister has been requested to bring a special bead and a prayer/blessing for the Mother.

When handed the string, the sister will share a story of her connection to the Mother, perhaps how they met, how long they have been friends, some challenges they have overcome or some funny embarrassing moments.

Positive and empowering birth stories can also be shared. This helps to create an intimate space and special moment. When she is ready, she will take a breath, place her bead to her heart and speak her blessing to the mother. The blessing is to focus on empowering the mother for a positive birth experience and initiation or deepening into motherhood.

When finished, she can blow on the bead to intone it with her breath and energy and then thread it onto the string. She then passes it on to the next woman, and so on and so forth, until it comes back to the Mother to tie off.

The finished piece will be an original one-of-a-kind piece of jewellery, which can be held by the birthing Mother during labour or incorporated into the birth space or altar to draw upon the strength and support from her inner circle of sisters.

Sacred Cord Ritual

If there is enough length, each woman in the circle can hold the beading string as it makes its way back to the mother, who completes the circle. She can then tie it off and cut each woman loose from the circle, leaving enough string to create the anchoring thread. Otherwise, this can be a separate ritual where the mother-to-be ties red string onto the wrist or ankle of her inner circle sisters, and once the news of the baby's arrival, the sister is then able to remove the string any way she chooses and prepare her own sacred ceremony to welcome baby.

The string symbolises the *womb grid* and the invisible web that weaves all women together in solidarity and sisterhood! It also represents the baby's umbilical cord and, much like that of an umbilical cord, this invisible energetic cord connects the mother with her sisters woven into her inner circle of support.

In the days leading up to the birth, any time one of the inner circle sisters looks at her string, she can send prayers and love to mother and baby. It helps to keep people connected and is a strong, supportive energetic container to protect the *birth field*.

Birth Candle Ritual

All women present have a sheet of beeswax each. They share stories of positive birthing experiences, stories and offer blessings and prayers.

One by one, they add their layer of beeswax to create a rolled pillar candle, which is then gifted to the Mother. It can also be decorated with string from the other ceremonies, or perhaps each woman is given a length of string to share their blessing, a positive affirmation or a word and then wrap it around the finished candle.

Alternatively, messages and blessings can be written on paper and rolled with the candle. The candle can be left plain or dressed with essential oils and majickal herbs. Once the birthing mother feels she is in early or active labour, she can light the birth candle that will illuminate the birthing space with all the prayers and blessings bestowed upon her.

Henna

Henna is traditionally known in India as 'mendhi' and protects the womb and baby from outside energies. You can hire a professional, which I feel is best, to do a full belly sitting whilst mama is pampered, or you can buy a DIY kit and have guests add a line of henna on the mother's belly.

You can get templates to help create beautiful lines. Be mindful that a full belly piece can take a couple of hours. S great way to offer this is if all guests chip in to hire someone so that the expectant mother can have her belly adorned uninterrupted and can have it on display (if she chooses) on the day of her blessing ceremony.

Water/Flower Blessing with Essential oils

Women gather and prepare a bowl of distilled water and using soothing essential oils, like lavender, sandalwood, frankincense, jasmine, rose, etc, then add a drop each, with a prayer or blessing. This main brew can then be stored in amber spritz bottles and used as a facial mist or room spray by the mother.

Fire Ritual

All women gather together to write down their fears and insecurities about labour and birth. These are then offered into sacred fire to release the energy and help to cleanse and purify the *birth field* from any discordant energy or anxiety. The ash can then be scattered on the Earth with love.

Placenta Bag

If having a lotus birth, women can help to make a placenta bag. There are many sewing patterns online and it can be a fun and crafty afternoon bonding activity. The bag is designed to be waterproof and makes for easy breastfeeding and recovery as the bag is soft and can be kept alongside the baby until the umbilical cord naturally detaches.

Flower Crown

All guests bring some flowers, which can be used in the centre of the sacred circle, becoming imbued with the spiritual energy of the ceremony and then crafted into a flower crown at the end. After adorning the new mother with her crown, take photos for keepsakes. If there are enough flowers, perhaps everyone wears a flower crown for a group photo.

Affirmations Flags

You can purchase *'fat quarters'** from your local sewing supply or craft shop. These can then be cut to an ideal size and painted with fabric paint to create affirmation flags for the birth space. Alternatively, guests could create their own beautiful artwork with positive and uplifting quotes, mantras or words that can help to uplift and inspire the new mother to feel confident in birthing her baby safely. Please refer to the Affirmations in the Birth Warrior chapter.

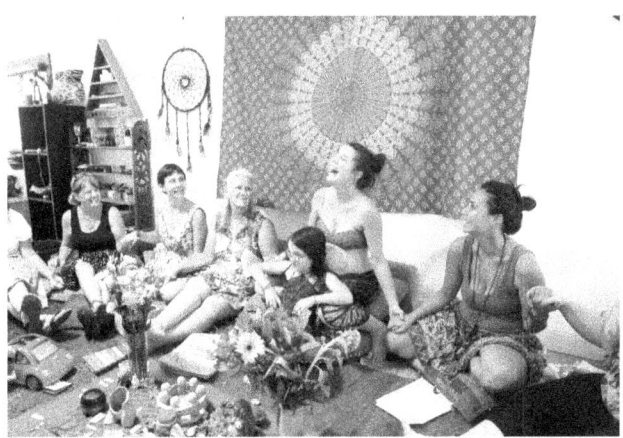

My 2016 Mother Blessing ceremony was facilitated by one of my Sacred Circle students, Kim (pictured right).

---

* Using the Australian metric system, a fat quarter is a piece of fabric generally used in quilting that measures approximately 50x54 cm

Run Sheet for a Mother Blessing Event

The Mother Blessings ceremony is facilitated by someone other than the expectant Mother. It can be someone close to her or a hired professional. Below is a run sheet of a simple mother blessings ceremony which you can use and adjust as you see fit.

- Guests arrive.
- Tea and light refreshments + mingling time. Ensure everyone is fed before you start the ceremony, this will allow for more focus, as sometimes the rituals take longer than expected.
- Call to circle
- Smoke cleansing with either local dried aromatic and majickal herbs, culturally significant smudging or an aromatic spritz upon entry.
- Guests place sacred offerings onto an altar if needed. If you want a gift table, keep this separate, to the side and out of the way of the circle space.
- Opening Circle, weaving the inner circle of sisters. Welcome everyone to the space, acknowledgement for traditional custodians of the land and ancestors.
- Nurturing for mama begins, think foot bath, massage etc.
- Share positive and uplifting birth stories
- Rituals (choose from the list above)
- Close Sacred Circle
- Before guests leave, discuss a Meal Train* and develop an action plan for post-birth support. A meal train is a fantastic way to support new parents in bonding and connecting deeply with their newborn during the imprinting stages. If everyone is clear on the mother's dietary restrictions, then

---

* A Meal Train is an organised way for friends and family to deliver home-cooked meals or groceries during the postpartum stage to help support and care for the new Mother and family.

meals can be prepared and frozen in advance. These are such a gift of love and so helpful in the early days.
- Food+ fun
- Close

Naming Ceremony

A NAME IS MORE than just a label; it's a profound gift of identity, a symbol of belonging and an energetic signature for the Soul to manifest and express itself through. A name is a foundational aspect of human identity, a vibrational anchor in which we are called home to ourselves with sound. It is not merely a string of letters; it's a sacred symbolic gift that carries the essence of who we are and who we aspire to be.

The act of naming is life-affirming and holds profound psychological and spiritual implications. It shapes our sense of belonging and connection to our lineage, culture, country and spiritual energy. Moreover, a name can influence our self-perception and behaviour, serving as a guiding force throughout our lives.

When a name is dreamed in, spoken with intention and bestowed with love and reverence, it becomes a source of empowerment reinforcing one's sense of identity, belonging and purpose. By formally introducing someone to their name within a ceremonial context, we honour their existence and acknowledge their place within their family, community and the world.

Across cultures, naming ceremonies are facilitated through rituals and traditions that imbue the occasion with spiritual meaning, protection and blessings. From recitations of prayers and blessings to the lighting of candles, smoking of aromatic herbs, the sprinkling of water or the tying of symbolic cords, these rituals symbolise the child's entry into the community and invoke blessings for their health, happiness and prosperity. Family members, elders, and community leaders often play integral roles in the ceremony, offering wisdom, guidance and support for the child's journey.

. . .

THE DIVERSITY of naming ceremonies reflects the richness of human culture and the adaptability of tradition to changing times. Some Aboriginal communities hold special ceremonies to introduce newborns to their skin names and kinship groups formally. These ceremonies often involve rituals, songs, dances and prayers conducted by elders or community leaders to bless the child and welcome them to country (which is not separate from self) and into the community.

IN CATHOLIC TRADITIONS, baptism is a common naming ceremony where a child is officially welcomed into the faith community. Water symbolises purification and rebirth during the ceremony and the child is given a Christian name. Godparents or sponsors are often chosen to guide the child's spiritual journey.

IN HINDU TRADITION, the Namkarana ceremony ('Naam' and 'Karan' mean 'name' and 'form') is performed to name the newborn child. The name is typically chosen based on astrological considerations, auspicious timing or familial significance. During the ceremony, prayers and rituals invoke blessings for the child's health, happiness and prosperity.

MANY NATIVE AMERICAN tribes have their own unique naming ceremonies that honour the child's connection to nature, ancestors and community. These ceremonies often involve rituals such as smudging with sacred herbs, drumming, singing and the offering of traditional gifts. The child's name may be chosen based on visions, dreams or spiritual guidance.

AMONG THE MĀORI people of New Zealand, the Whakapapa naming ceremony is a traditional practice emphasising the child's ancestral connections and spiritual lineage. During the ceremony, elders recite genealogical chants, share ancestors' stories and bestow upon the child their Maori name, which connects them to the land and the *mana* (universal energy) of place.

Whether rooted in cultural tradition, religion or spirituality, naming ceremonies serve as powerful expressions of love, identity and belonging, which remind us all of the beauty, significance and sanctity of one of life's most precious gifts; the gift of a name.

Simple Naming Ceremony Run Sheet

- Welcome and Introduction.
- Guests begin to arrive and are greeted by hosts.
- The officiant welcomes guests and introduces the purpose of the gathering.
- Guests are invited to find their seats.
- Parents and the baby enter the ceremony space accompanied by music.
- The officiant welcomes everyone to the naming ceremony and sets the tone for the event.
- Parents share the chosen name of their child with the gathered guests.
- Family members, friends or elders offer blessings and well wishes for the child's future. Handwritten blessings can be kept for the coming-of-age ceremony later.
- Parents participate in a symbolic ritual to mark the significance of the naming ceremony (e.g., lighting a candle, burying the placenta, planting a tree or tying a symbolic cord).
- The officiant offers closing remarks, expressing gratitude to everyone for joining the celebration.
- Guests are invited to a reception to enjoy refreshments and continue celebrating with the family.
- Guests offer their congratulations to the family and begin to depart

PART III- THE PRIMAL WILD
NAVIGATING THE SPIRITUAL DIMESIONS OF LABOUR AND BIRTH

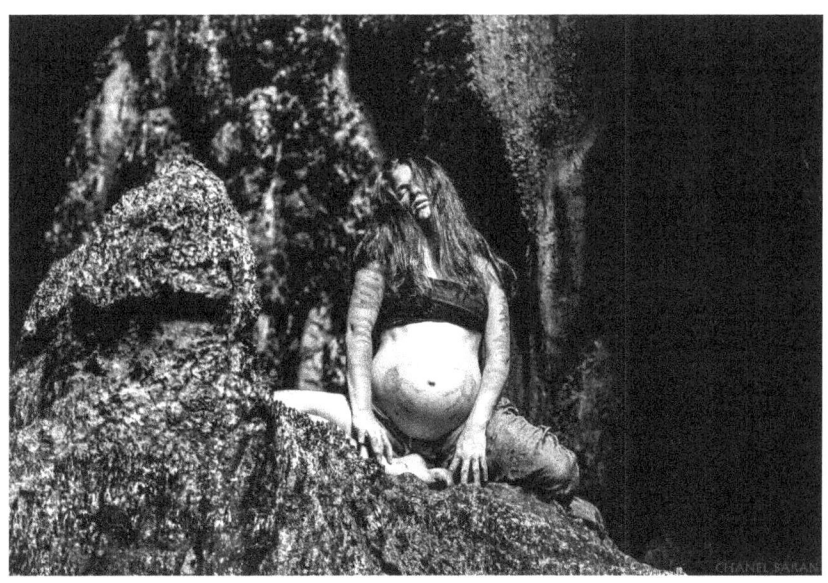

"Woman is the radiance of God. She is not a creature. She is the creator." -Rumi

11

PREPARE TO BIRTH
ACTIVATING THE BIRTH SPIRAL

"Birth is not only about making babies. Birth is about making mothers-strong, competent, capable mothers who trust themselves and know their inner strength."
— Barbara Katz Rothman

Birth is not something that happens to you and your baby, it is something that you both facilitate together. The birth of a baby means the birth of a Mother and as you continue to connect with your baby; have conversations about the nature of birth, express your desires and how you would like it to unfold. This engagement helps to create a bond and understanding that strengthens your journey together as a team.

You can begin to program your mind early on to manifest an empowered birthing experience, whether it's an undisturbed natural birth or a planned medical birth. As a creatrix, you hold that power! However, it's important to recognise that you cannot control *The Great Mystery*. A significant part of the process is to keep focusing on the type of birth you desire, how you want to feel, and how you want your baby to feel, and then release the outcome. The 'how' is not up to you.

Your focus needs to be on maintaining your presence with your body and baby throughout the journey as it unfolds. Being unattached to the outcome grants you the freedom to open up to incredible possibilities beyond the scope of your current knowledge. It also means that in the worst-case scenario, you will still be there, in the moment completely present and walking it step by step with your baby. Fixating on the perfect birth will not serve you because there is no such thing.

Birth is raw, messy and dynamic. Being present and mindful allows you to respond to the ebb and flow of labour and birth with grace, Embracing each moment as it comes and trusting in your body's wisdom and your baby's instincts. By cultivating this mindset, you create receptivity to the natural flow of the birthing process.

Ultimately, the birth journey is about surrendering to the unknown and embracing the transformative power it holds. It is about being open to the experience however it may unfold and finding strength in the connection between you and your baby. As you prepare for birth, remember you are not alone in this journey. You are co-creating a new life and in doing so, you are discovering new depths of your own being.

RECOMMENDED BOOKS:

- **Birth Without Violence**- Frederik Leboyer
- **Voices From The Womb**- Michael Gabriel
- **Ten Moons**- Jane Hardwicke Collings
- **Birth with Confidence**- Rhea Dempsey
- **Down to Earth Birth Book**- Jenny Blyth
- **Spiritual Midwifery**- Ina May Gaskin
- **The Fourth Trimester**- Kimberly Ann Johnson

Websites:

- **Spinningbabies.com**
- **TheMylesCircuit.com**

Ripen and Retreat

At around 33 weeks, it's time to switch off from the noise, chaos and drama of the external and digital world. In my opinion, this is not the time for social media, you do not owe anyone anything right now. Your little womb fruit is ripening, and these last weeks will feel like they are dragging on. Engage yourself in activities that nourish your Spirit and fill your cup. It is important to allow yourself to go inwards and put the final preparations into action for complete mind-body-soul synchronisation. Optimal birthing energy is one of open receptivity and expansion of energy. You can not do this fully when stressed, or your nervous system is dysregulated and overstimulated. This is the time for peace, joy and bliss, a time to fully immerse in the experience of the ripening stages of pregnancy and retreat from the external world so that you can amplify the signals from your internal world, allowing you to sync deeper with your inner wisdom and listening to your baby.

AROUND 38 WEEKS, if possible, I suggest this be a 'no contact' zone… earlier if you carry multiples. Guard your energetic space. Make sure you have completed all your ceremonies and photoshoots. I say this because, at this stage, your baby is fully developed and ready to go any day. You must prioritise rest, relaxation, oxytocin production and connecting with your partner and birth support team. Your life and identity are about to radically transform as you transition from *Maiden into Mother.*

Give yourself the space to embody your wild Maiden energy, allow this part of yourself to be witnessed and expressed and grieve this time of transition if you need to, so that you are ready to cross the threshold into motherhood. There is big psychic work happening. You are about to cross dimensions, this is a time for grounding and focused intent. A time to come home to your power and your majick.

Linger in this sacred moment; there is nowhere else you need to be, and you may not be gifted this opportunity again. Be with it. All of it. You've come so far, your body has changed so much, and big work is ahead- that is why it is commonly called labour!

Activating the Birth Spiral

The spiral is incredibly sacred and is one of the most ancient symbols known to man and fundamentally links us to the movement and expression of creation energy. It manifests from the micro to the macrocosm, evident in the structure of DNA, the spiral pattern of electrons around atoms and the vast spiralling structures of galaxies and celestial bodies. Representing the dynamic process of becoming, the spiral symbolises cyclic energy across time and space from the infinitesimal to the infinite. Birth marks the beginning of a new spiral, creating a path for consciousness to experience itself through the cycles of life, as a fractal. Thus, the *Birth Spiral* poignantly underscores the interconnectedness of all things and the perpetual cycle of creation and renewal in life's universal dance with *The Great Mystery*.

When a Mother is safe and has the opportunity to connect with her primal body wisdom, she will naturally spiral her hips with a gentle movement. This spiralling helps to bring the baby down into the pelvis and working with the breath will allow her to move beyond the intense sensations in her body. The birth spiral also represents the internal journey of a Mother as she activates the energetic field around her to cross dimensions and bring her baby through. As labour progresses, there's a natural turning inward, focusing on primal instincts, sensations and emotions. This inward journey mirrors spiralling deeper into oneself, shedding emotional layers for acknowledgment and release. Journeying with the spiral, you can reach back in time and access a reservoir of ancestral wisdom that links you to all those who have birthed before.

To activate the *Birth Spiral*, intentionally engage your body in a circular motion through dance, spiralling the hips or rocking back and forth, bringing your awareness to the energy that wants to move with and through you. You are a conduit for creation energy, a sacred portal ready to open from one world into the other so that you can receive your beautiful baby. Bring your joyous energy into your birth space, sing, dance, rejoice and call to your child.

In the last few days of pregnancy, focus your awareness on the sensation of stillness and then once you feel rooted in this stillness, bring some gentle spiralling motion into your body through your hips. Whether you're standing, on all fours or sitting on a birth ball, bring all your awareness into your pelvis. Breathe deeply and attune your senses to the cosmic energy around you and in the very fabric of your cells. You may start to feel warmth or a buzzing sensation around you as you amplify the spiritual energy of your birth space. If you're a visual person, you may even begin to see a vortex of spiralling energy above you. Activating the *Birth Spiral* signals the universe that you are ready for your baby to descend and engage birth, ready for a new spiral to begin.

Preparing Your Birth Space

If you're preparing to give birth at home, harness your nesting energy to cleanse and prepare your space. Begin this process around 34-38 weeks, creating a sanctuary that resonates with your birthing intentions and provides a nurturing environment for you and your baby.

Start bringing in ceremonial tools that hold meaning and power for you. These might include candles, blessing ceremony beads, a birth tub, shamanic ritual tools, talismans, affirmation flags and inspiring images. When the surges begin, light your birthing candle to signal the commencement of this sacred journey. Fill your space with music and movement. Sing your favourite songs or the *soul song* that connects you to your baby. Engage in dance and movement to activate your pelvis and hips, using spiralling and circular motions to encourage openness and flow.

Spend time in your birth space reading, meditating, making love and connecting with your partner. Ensure that the energy in this space remains positive and supportive. In the lead-up to birth, if your partner's energy is off, do not welcome them into the space until they are emotionally regulated and rooted in their presence. Protect this sanctuary, allowing no one to infiltrate it unless invited by you. This is your domain. Use this space for healing and addressing any unresolved emotions. Clear away any mother/father wounds and engage in shadow work to create a harmonious birthing experience. Practice emotional alchemy through *Womb Song*, EFT (Emotional Freedom Techniques), kinetic breathwork, and mindset work to transform any lingering fears or anxieties.

IDENTIFY any residual fear or anxiety you may have and give voice to it so you can release the emotional charge and take your power back. Become familiar with birthing positions and how you will move around your birth space- adjust furniture or set up little stations to support a comfortable labour, birth and integration time.

If you choose to give birth in the hospital, see if you can book a time to see the room or birth suite to become familiar with the setting. Walk the space, hum the space. Speak to your baby and familiarise yourself with the sights and sounds so it can feel like a temporary home. Ask any questions about medical equipment so you are not intimidated by what is in the room. This will allow you to switch your mind off during labour.

Remember, wherever you go, the spiral goes, too!

Conscious Birth Plan

First things first... be prepared for your birth plan to go right out the window! Seriously, it doesn't matter how much time you invest in creating the 'perfect' plan, the reality is that your birth may not go to plan, and this is totally ok! The most important part about the plan is what you will and will not consent to.

Preparing a birth plan serves the purpose of getting you in the mindset to think about what might happen and how you can be prepared for it. Creating a birth plan is more about having a way for you to have clarity in communication about your needs before the big day. When you begin labour, your prefrontal cortex will begin to shut down as you access the primal mamillion part of the brain and it's important you are undisturbed during this process to be able to trust your body to do what it needs to do, naturally. Having a birth plan and delegating someone to advocate for your needs will support you to focus on doing what you need to do, going within, to access your primal wisdom and birth your baby. You want to avoid unnecessary questions that will snap you out of this deep embodiment experience of labour, especially if you're prone to overthinking. So it's best to talk it all through beforehand.

Things to Think About

- Where do you want to have your baby?
- Do you want access to pain relief? If so, what kind?
- What do you want to avoid, and what is an absolute non-negotiable?
- Who do you want with you as a birth support partner?
- If you need extra assistance, who are you comfortable having in your space? - Partner, mother, children, doula, friends and other relatives.
- Do you want your birth support to be present all the time?
- Would you prefer to be left alone?
- Do you want to be spoken to during labour?
- Do you want to be touched? Know your boundaries and that it is ok to have them.
- What are the roles and responsibilities of your birth support?
- Do you want immediate skin-to-skin contact?
- If you are in the hospital and certain interventions need to take place, do you want your support people present, or do they leave the room and come back?
- Who will be your trusted voice to speak on your behalf if needed? This person needs to be someone connected to you and what you wish for your birthing experience- they might need to speak about pain relief, intervention, internal examinations, etc.
- What positions do you want to use to birth your baby?
- What birthing aids will you need to help support you?
- Do you want a water birth?
- Who is responsible for preparing the water and managing the temperature?
- Do you prefer different lighting?
- If in a hospital, is it possible to turn the lights off and have a lamp?

- How would you like to create your Sacred Birthing space?
- Do you want a music player, diffuser, candles, prayer flags, etc?
- What music would you like to listen to?
- Who is responsible for starting the playlist?
- Do you want to cut the cord, delayed cord clamping or lotus birth? Do you want to keep the placenta?
- How can all of this be supported if you have an emergency medical birth?
- What are your non-negotiables?

Medical Intervention- What If's

- If your homebirth turns into an emergency, who is responsible for calling for help and getting an ambulance?
- If it reaches the point, would you prefer to have an episiotomy or natural tear?
- What are your options for healing the wound?
- If your labour stalls, how will you help to progress?
- What herbs would you like to use? Do you have them?
- Do you want your caregiver (if any) to administer anything to help?
- Do you want to wait to transfer? Who makes the call?
- How do you feel about induction?
- How long are you comfortable with being 'post-term'
- Would you agree to induction? What methods, natural or synthetic?
- How do you feel about internal examinations to check for dilation?
- What about fetal monitoring or insertion of catheter, saline drip, etc?
- Under what circumstances would you agree to a cesarean? - exhaustion, emergency only etc
- What is the protocol for cesarean, can you stay awake?
- What is the bonding time with the baby?

- How can you ensure you and your baby are together for important bonding and imprinting?
- Will your partner be present with you?
- How can you support yourself post-birth to recover from surgery?
- How can you help to speed up wound healing and recovery?
- If you cannot give consent, who will have the authority to speak for you on your behalf?

It is important to go over your birth plan with anyone involved with the birth before 36 weeks so that everyone is on the same page and clear of their roles and responsibilities so that they can also be prepared. It is important to have adequate information for informed decision-making and consent.

Preparing yourself with clear communication will help to eliminate any subconscious fears you may have around birth and the what-ifs. When dealing with the medical establishment, know that they work for you and that you have the power of authority over your body and your baby.

Always ask, *"What's it for, and is it necessary?"*

This way, you can be provided with relevant information and can make your decision accordingly. Depending on where you live, you may need to have someone who can help be your backbone to eliminate any pressure or bullying tactics to pressure you into making decisions you are uncomfortable with.

Homebirth and Freebirth Preparation

What you need:

- Clear and comfortable birthing space. Dark or dim light is best.
- Birth pool or access to bathtub if you are planning to water birth.
- Hoses with proper connections (One birth I attached to the showerhead, the other to the washing machine taps as I

birthed in a different space. You can purchase fittings from the hardware store in the plumbing section. Ensure you run the hose through with a good flush of water if it is brand new, otherwise, you could risk infection.)

- Bucket for spew/excrement.
- Strainer- aka 'pooper scooper' *Remember: The solution to pollution is dilution.*
- Bath thermometer to gauge the temperature of the birth pool water. You want to keep it at body temp- 36 degrees Celsius.
- Any props for labour, birth ball, small stool, cushions/bolsters for support, etc.
- Any sacred talismans or objects to put into your birthing space that helps to anchor the spiritual energy. This includes candles, oils, cards, affirmations, blessing ceremony beads, prayer flags, etc. I would caution you not to put too much stuff in there- you do not want to create too much stimulus as it can prevent you from dropping into the primal internal realms.
- Towels- lots of them, preferably light in colour so that you can monitor blood loss. You can call upon friends and family for old towels or grab some from a local thrift shop.
- Face washers for during labour that can be used to pat you down, keep you cool.
- Ice to keep hydrated; you can also freeze some of your favourite juice.
- High-grade Manuka honey for postpartum recovery and keeping your blood sugar level up, if you don't feel like eating.
- Incontinence sheets or a splash blanket, if you can access them, are great for the afterbirth bonding time, so you don't have to worry about bleeding through bedding or furniture.
- A bowl to birth/store placenta. I used a stainless steel bowl.
- Placenta bag, rice steamer or container to store placenta if you are lotus birthing.
- Fresh, clean towels to cover yourself and your baby.
- If it's cold, a warm wheat pack or hot water bottle makes it easier to warm up towels.

- A Sacred vessel to catch first blood to use in ritual.
- Music playlist sorted, ready and tested.
- Essential oils suitable for birthing (lavender, clary sage, etc.) and diffuser.
- Motherwort and Shepherds Purse tincture- 10 drops straight under the tongue after birth.
- Ambulance on standby or notify the local midwife/ hospital about your plans so that on the off chance that something happens, they know to expect you.
- Maternity pads or incontinence pants for your postpartum lochia. They look like adult nappies but are so awesome for catching all the uterine clots in the days following birth

BIRTH IS a delicate balance of life and death. The safety and comfort of the Mother are of utmost importance, although sometimes things don't go according to your birth plan. There are many mindset coaches that espouse having a bag packed goes against manifesting the ideal birth- as it is creates fear and doubt on the outcome you are wanting to create. I call bullshit on this and think it is a dangerous form of spiritual bypassing. The mature approach is to be prepared, despite your best intentions and mindset practices. Life has a way of happening, regardless of how prepared we are, so have a bag packed with a change of clothes, toiletries and phone charger just in case. The nature of birth is a grand mystery. I advise entering this space maturely and covering all the "what-ifs" in advance. This way, you can fully surrender to the presence of your initiation with acceptance of how it all unfolds.

Birth Affirmations

If you feel called to have affirmations in your space, it might be a great opportunity to explore your creative side and turn them into artwork. Feel free to use any of the prompts below or draw inspiration and create your own.

If you find that your mind continually dances with anxiety and fear, the affirmations can be a positive way to train your brain and create a healthy and strong mindset to prepare to bring your baby Earthside.

Feel free to use, modify, or personalise the following affirmations to suit your journey.

- My body knows exactly what to do to birth my baby.
- I trust in my ability to birth with strength and confidence.
- Each surge brings my baby closer to me.
- I am safe, I am supported, and I am loved.
- My cervix opens easily and naturally.
- I surrender to the natural rhythm of my body and my baby.
- I release any fear and tension, allowing my body to relax.
- I am surrounded by love and encouragement.
- My baby is perfectly positioned for birth.
- I breathe in calmness and breathe out tension.
- I embrace the power of my contractions, knowing they bring me closer to meeting my baby.
- I am connected to generations of women who have birthed before me.
- My body is designed for this miraculous journey of birth.
- With each contraction, I visualise my baby moving down and into position.
- I am patient and present, allowing labour to unfold in its own time.
- I trust the wisdom of my body and my baby.
- I welcome each sensation as a sign of progress and strength.
- I am capable, I am strong, and I am ready.
- I release any doubts and embrace my inner power.
- I am a fierce, loving, and determined mother.
- I surround myself with positive energy and affirmations.
- I am supported by my birthing team and loved ones.
- I visualise my cervix opening like a blossoming flower.
- I listen to my body's cues and respond with love and trust.
- I trust the process of birth and surrender to its wisdom.

- Each surge brings me closer to holding my baby in my arms.
- I release any tension in my body and mind, allowing for a smooth and easy birth.
- I am filled with gratitude for the opportunity to birth my baby.
- My body is capable of miracles, and birthing my baby is one of them.
- I am surrounded by a circle of love and support, both seen and unseen.
- I visualise my pelvis opening wide to welcome my baby's journey earthside.
- I am at peace with whatever path my birth journey takes.
- I trust my instincts and intuition to guide me through labour and birth.
- I am calm, I am centred, and I am ready to give birth to my baby.
- I am a strong and capable woman.
- I am a fierce and protective birthing mama.
- My body is strong and built to birth with ease.
- I am in complete control of my body and mind.
- I trust my instincts to know what I need for my labour.
- I release and flow with the energy of my surge.
- I am confident in my ability to birth my baby.
- I am a fearless mama.
- I am a warrior mama.
- I am fearless.
- I am powerful.
- I allow myself to surrender and ride the surges with my breath.
- I can breathe my baby down and through.
- I trust that my baby will help to facilitate the perfect birth for its soul's journey.
- The strength of my surge symbolises my strength as a woman.
- I am encoded with incredible primal wisdom that I will access during birth.

- I am guided by Spirit/God/Goddess/Creation to be a bridge between worlds.
- I am a portal of life and love.
- The power and intensity of my surges/contractions will lead me to my power and resilience.
- My body knows how to give birth to my baby calmly and peacefully.
- I am deeply grounded in my ability to birth my baby safely.
- I am connected to the wisdom of all mothers who have birthed before me.
- I take my place in the grand cosmic wheel of time.
- I am at peace and surrender to the great mystery of birth.
- I am alive and deeply connected to the Divine will of creation.
- I connect with my voice and speak my truth clearly.
- I am honoured and cherished for my role as a conscious birthing mother.
- My birth will be a profoundly spiritual initiation.
- I step into motherhood with an open heart.
- My birth will be exactly as it needs to be.
- I can and will have an empowered birth.
- My birth will be a deeply spiritual experience.
- I am ready to receive Sacred Feminine Wisdom.
- I am supported by ALL birthing mothers.
- I am connected to my voice and my heart.
- I am ready.
- May the energy of Birth guide me.
- I see my baby in the perfect position for birthing.
- I am in complete control of my body and mind.
- I am deeply connected to my baby and our journey together.
- I am capable of handling whatever comes my way during birth.
- Each contraction brings me closer to meeting my baby.
- I am surrounded by love and positive energy.
- My body is perfectly designed for birthing my baby.
- I trust the natural process of birth to unfold beautifully.
- I welcome each surge with an open heart and mind.

- I am supported by a team that believes in my strength and ability.
- My baby's birth will be a sacred and transformative experience.
- I embrace the sensations of labour as signs of progress and power.
- I am deeply connected to the wisdom of my ancestors who birthed before me.
- I am filled with courage and determination as I give birth to my baby.
- I release any tension in my body and surrender to the birthing process.
- I am surrounded by the loving presence of my birth companions.
- I trust my body's innate ability to birth my baby with ease.
- I am a vessel of life and love, bringing new life into the world.
- I welcome each surge with gratitude and acceptance.
- I am strong, capable, and resilient in any challenge.
- My body instinctively knows how to give birth to my baby safely.
- I am empowered to make choices that align with my birthing preferences.
- I am connected to the strength and wisdom of all birthing women throughout history.
- I surrender to the flow of birth, trusting in its divine timing.
- I am surrounded by a supportive and loving birthing environment.
- I trust my intuition to guide me through each moment of labour and birth.
- I am worthy of a positive and empowering birth experience.
- I am filled with love and excitement as I prepare to meet my baby.
- I am grateful for the opportunity to experience the miracle of birth.

Birth Songs

Confident Mother

I am a strong and confident Mother
I birth my baby with ease.
I trust my body as I ride these surges
I step into the Mystery.
I am connected, I am whole
I remember what I already know.
Woven into life's grand tapestry
The power of creation resides in me.
I am a strong and confident mother and
I birth my baby with ease.

FEET on the Earth Birth Chant

With My feet on the Earth I birth I birth
With my feet on the Earth I birth (x4)
I am connected. I am embodied
I am strong in the Primal Wild.
I am a mother opening
to love, Divine
With My feet on the Earth I birth I birth
With my feet on the Earth I birth (x2)
I am connected. I am embodied
I am strong in the Primal Wild.
I am a mother listening
To the wisdom of my womb.
With My feet on the Earth I birth I birth
With my feet on the Earth I birth (x2)
I am connected I am embodied
I am strong in the primal wild
I am a mother opening
to love, Divine.
With My feet on the Earth I birth I birth
With my feet on the Earth I birth (x2)

. . .

GRANDMOTHER WISDOM
  Grandmother wisdom guide me,
  Hold me, carry me.
  Grandmother wisdom help me see,
  the truth from fear, bring me clarity.
  Grandmother wisdom help me understand,
  the language of birth please hold my hand.
  Grandmother Wisdom please show me,
  how to birth my baby.
  I trust in your sacred ways

SURRENDER
  I am opening, Surrendering.
  The great mystery consumes me whole.
  I am opening, Surrendering.
  The Primal Wild takes me on the inside.
  I walk alone into the unknown.
  I walk with grace until I meet your face.
  With your head to my breast we can now rest.

MAIDEN TO MOTHER
  It's time for me to go now,
  I can not come with you to this new place
  it's time to let go now
  integrate not erase.
  I will always be here, I will lay at your feet
  For you and I are one in the same
  And there will be seasons and reasons
  to call on me again.
  I will remind you to wander and wonder
  We will spin dance and sing
  we will laugh and celebrate

the majick that I bring
but it's time for me to go now
to lay down at your feet
as you become a mother
One i'm proud to meet
You've got important work to do
I'll walk beside you with grace
this is not goodbye
integrate not erase.

Safe Passage

I move like the tide
the birth spiral opens wide
Baby in my heart
baby in my womb
baby I will come get you
and breathe you through
safe passage to me, baby
safe passage to you.

12

THE SACRED SPIRAL
THE ETERNAL DANCE OF BIRTH AND DEATH

> "Life is the journey between the darkness of the womb
> and darkness of the grave."
> -Ala Bashir

Life as we know it is ephemeral, constantly changing and rearranging. You only have to look towards Nature to find this wisdom on constant display and considering we are part of Nature's great wide web of creation, we too, have our seasons. Life and death are two sides of the same coin. The dance of the sacred spiral. Each birth symbolises an impending death and each death, signifies the birth of something new. Death is a Sacred Rite of Passage we share with every living thing, one that no one can avoid. We are all given a lifetime, the duration and quality of which varies.

Contemporary culture is so afraid of death to the extent that interventions infiltrate this often natural process to preserve life at all costs, even if it is quality of life for an individual and the amplification of their suffering... atleast they're alive, right? Personal choice in this regard is considered taboo and shameful. Think of abortion, euthanasia and suicide, for example.

When you are seeding life within your womb, whether by choice or not, you enter into a sacred dance, a cosmic ebb and flow of *the Great Mystery*. There will always be two outcomes: birth and death. It is binary, and we can not escape this reality. This is the medicine of the womb, the light and the dark. The more you are willing to surrender to the mystery as it unfolds, the easier it will be to process the myriad potentials around you and the choices and realities you may face now and in the future. Choices that may differ over time as your circumstances and beliefs change.

You can never truly know the future, so compassion is key for yourself and others. There are many women and families around the world faced with incredibly harsh realities, ones they never thought they'd be in and yet there they are. The intricacies of life present us with opportunities for unfathomable joy and grief. All beautiful and necessary.

As uncomfortable as some of this may be, it is part of the sacred dance when you realise you are connected to something bigger than yourself, a divine timeline of your destiny unfolding in all its beautiful mess. Sometimes you get lucky, sometimes you don't! Sometimes, our experiences can be unfair as life does not discriminate on social or economic status, religious beliefs, or how 'good' you are. Sometimes shit happens and you have to deal with it as best you can, but death, well, death is coming for us all and it is to be revered, not feared.

Facing Death

There are so many variables and potential realities beyond your control. I have found that coming to peace and acceptance with death has allowed me to be more present in my body and the whole precious journey of pregnancy and birth and life in general.

As a young girl, one of my first spiritual initiations was processing my own mortality. At the tender age of 10, I had no compass to help me navigate through crippling anxiety as I questioned the purpose of life because from my perspective, the moment you are born, you begin to die. Death was the ultimate endpoint. Game over. This spun me into an existential crisis that lead me to seek and explore *Gnosis**.

It has been through the experiences of love, deep loss and emotional alchemy practices that I've received the medicine of death, which imbues life with meaning. We all have unique life experiences, each with different durations. With the understanding that education leads to empowerment, let's examine the facts to address subconscious fears.

In 2017, According to the Australian Bureau of Statistics, the infant mortality rate (birth to 1 year) was 3.3 infant deaths per 1,000 live births. in the USA, it was 5.7 infant deaths per 1,000 live births (2017), and in the UK, it was 3.76 infant deaths per 1,000 live births (2015). Remember that these statistics speak to the timeframe of a live birth to the first 49 days postpartum. These statistics will vary for each country, though the highest rates are often seen in countries with lower socio-economic status and limited access to resources and safe hygiene practices. In 2021, The maternal mortality rate in Australia was 5.8 deaths per 100,000 women giving birth, with the most common causes being cardiovascular, sepsis, non-obstetric haemorrhage and suicide. [1]

From a space of non-attachment, we gift ourselves the ability to surrender to *the Great Mystery* completely and to trust the bigger picture that will be revealed to us in due course.

As a birthing Mother, your role is to prepare yourself physically, emotionally and spiritually for your initiation, to nurture and facilitate the environment that supports life to the best of your ability, to know that even in the event of death, you were present with the gift of life inside and outside of you.

Birth can have many inherent risks and the unknown can be quite frightening. Still, when a woman is left undisturbed and is nurtured in a way that fosters a deep connection to her primordial state of being, she has the ability to tap into her primal wisdom to birth her baby safely. This includes her choice of when, where and how she gives birth, who she allows into her space and what intervention is necessary whilst

---

* Gnosis is the common greek word for knowledge. It also represents intuitive knowledge and spiritual truth.

always retaining her autonomy. In this way, the Spirit of the Mother remains whole and connected.

Therapeutic Miscarriage and Abortion

In Australia, approximately 25% of pregnancies are unplanned, of which one-third end in abortion, although there is no data on precise numbers. South Australia is one of the only states to collect and publish their abortion data; over 90% of abortions in that state occur in the first trimester each year, with less than 2% occurring after 20 weeks gestation. The majority of post-20-week procedures are provided for fetal reasons.

Early medical abortion, also known as therapeutic or chemical miscarriage, is a less invasive alternative to surgical abortion for pregnancies up to nine weeks gestation. Using the drugs mifepristone and misoprostol is more cost-effective than the surgical option. It is a safe option to complete at home, with a follow-up from a healthcare professional.

Worldwide, one in four pregnancies end in termination. Access to safe abortion is one of the most heated topics around the world and the continual moral, ethical and religious debate often distorts the true ramifications of limiting access to safe and basic healthcare for women. Despite the legal status of abortion, women around the world will continue to seek this basic human right as they have done so in the past. Where there are strict laws, it will often lead women to seek unsafe abortions, which can put their health at risk. It is estimated that around 25 million unsafe abortions are completed each year.

Some of the complications women face from unsafe abortions are infection, injury and according to the World Health Organisation (WHO), it is the third leading cause of maternal deaths worldwide.

Other statistics[2] from the WHO include;

- Where abortion is legal and permitted on broad grounds, it is generally safe and where it is illegal in many circumstances, it is often unsafe. For example, in South Africa, the incidence of infection resulting from abortion decreased by 52% after the abortion law was liberalised in 1996

- Because the world's population is concentrated in Asia, most abortions occur there (26 million yearly); nine million of these take place in China.
- The average woman must use some form of effective contraception for at least 20 years if she wants to limit her family size to two children and 16 years if she wants four children.
- Worldwide, an estimated five million women are hospitalised each year for treatment of abortion-related complications, such as haemorrhage and sepsis.
- Complications due to unsafe abortion procedures account for an estimated 13% of maternal deaths worldwide, or 47,000 per year.
- Almost all abortion-related deaths occur in developing countries. The highest number occurs in Africa.

According to Amnesty International, The World Health Organisation also estimates that even if all contraceptive users used contraception perfectly in every sexual encounter, there would still be six million unintended pregnancies every year.

Navigating Loss: Finding Solace in Sensitive Spaces

The journey of motherhood is a unique tapestry woven with threads of joy, love and profound connection. Yet, it's also a path that can lead to moments of deep sorrow and heartache, particularly when faced with the devastating loss of a child or diagnosis of a disease, defect or disability. In these moments of heartache, it's vital to find spaces of solace to be with grief, to find a pathway to heal and regain your power and purpose.

Grief is a deeply personal and multifaceted experience and there is no right or wrong way to navigate it. Suppose you find yourself grappling with the loss of a child or the news of your child's disability, which impacts the quality of life and your identity as a mother. In that case, allowing yourself the space to feel and express your emotions is essential. Permit yourself to grieve in whatever way feels most authentic to you, whether through tears, anger, creativity or quiet reflection. Allow yourself to wail and scream at the injustice of this loss and the death of your hopes and dreams.

SIT with grief so that it can gift you its medicine. It is a master teacher if you allow yourself to surrender and listen deeply to the wisdom that comes from the stillness. Do not be afraid of this. They say grief is love with no place to land. Remember that your feelings are valid and seeking support and solace from loved ones, support groups, or professional counsellors is okay.

During profound loss, it can be incredibly difficult to find meaning or purpose in life. Regardless of the length or quality of your child's life, their presence leaves an indelible mark on your heart and soul. Take time to honour and celebrate this, embracing the love and joy they bring to your life, however fleeting it may be. Share stories, songs, art, photographs or mementos that capture the essence of your child's Spirit. By cherishing and honouring your child's legacy, you affirm the enduring bond of love that transcends earthly boundaries.

Grief is not linear, so take your time.

Many women find solace in seeking moments of beauty, connection and spiritual resonance amidst the pain. Consider exploring rituals or ceremonies that honour the life of your child or process the loss of hopes and dreams. By cherishing and honouring your baby's legacy, you affirm the profound impact of their brief but beautiful existence and also find acceptance of yourself as a Mother.

Nurturing Your Postpartum Body and Mind Amidst Grief

Navigating the complexities of grief while tending to the needs of your postpartum body requires an abundance of compassion and patience. In the tender aftermath of loss, it's crucial to prioritise nurturing your physical and emotional well-being with gentle kindness and understanding. Be mindful of the profound hormonal shifts that accompany birth, which can amplify feelings of sadness, anxiety, and fatigue.

Take time to honour your postpartum body, recognising its resilience and the sacred journey it has undertaken. Embrace practices that nourish and replenish your body, such as nourishing meals, gentle movement and restorative self-care rituals. Cultivate moments of stillness and reflection, allowing yourself to process and honour the depth of your emotions with tenderness and grace.

Reach out for support* [3] to deal with the emptiness or feelings of failure that may arise. This is a normal response to such loss but remember that feelings are not facts, so allow yourself the grace to feel your feelings without attaching or anchoring your identity to your loss. Let yourself wail.

Infant loss is a profound and heartbreaking journey, yet within the depths of your grief lie seeds of resilience, compassion and spiritual growth. As you navigate this tender path, remember that you are not alone. Many women have walked this path, quietly. Reach out for support, nurture your emotional and spiritual well-being and trust in the healing power of love to guide you through the darkest nights into the dawn of a new day. You may find solace in the sacred spaces of your heart, where the light of love eternally shines and the journey of Motherhood, in all its complexities, is honoured and revered with unwavering love.

The Power of Ceremony for Bereaved Mothers

In the quiet aftermath of loss, when the echoes of shattered dreams and broken hearts reverberate through the ether, the power of ceremony offers a healing balm. Humans crave rituals that allow us to process and make sense of our experiences, especially those steeped in profound heartbreak. Whether these ceremonies are shared with others or held in the intimate sanctum of one's heart, they grant us the space to acknowledge the magnitude of our suffering and seek pathways of acceptance and healing to move on.

. . .

---

* I've compiled a list of online resources to help access support in navigating loss, grief and disability in the endnotes section of the book.

END-OF-LIFE CEREMONIES SERVE A PROFOUND PURPOSE, particularly for mothers grappling with the loss of a child or the loss of hopes and dreams due to birth trauma, disability or other unforeseen circumstances. These ceremonies bridge the ethereal realm of what might have been and the stark reality of what is now. They provide a structured moment to pause, reflect and honour the life and potential that has been lost, whilst cultivating the way to acceptance and healing.

Being confronted with death or the loss of cherished dreams is an excruciating experience. The dreams of a Mother often extend far beyond tangible reality, encompassing hopes for the future, the potential of a child and the life that was envisioned for them. When these dreams are suddenly and irrevocably altered, the resulting emotional and psychological pain can be overwhelming.

Ceremonies offer a way to turn this pain into purpose. They allow bereaved mothers to channel their grief into a meaningful act of remembrance and transformation. By creating a sacred space to honour their loss, they can begin to find solace and a sense of closure. Whether a formal gathering with family and friends or a solitary ritual, the ceremony acknowledges the depth of the loss and the strength required to endure it. For mothers who have faced birth trauma or the challenges of raising a child with a disability, ceremonies can also be a source of empowerment and resilience. They provide an opportunity to mourn the loss of the idealised experience of motherhood and to celebrate the unique journey they are on. Through these rituals, mothers can find a community of support and understanding, recognising that they are not alone in their struggles, that they are seen, heard and held.

Ceremonies can act as a catalyst for seeking further support and resources. They open the door to conversations about grief, mental health and the need for professional help, encouraging mothers to reach out and connect with others who can provide guidance and companionship on their healing journey. Ultimately, the power of ceremony lies in its ability to honour the full spectrum of human experience. It allows bereaved mothers to give voice to their pain, acknowledge their loss and find a sense of peace and purpose amidst the chaos. Through the sacred act of ceremony, they can begin to weave a new narrative that honours their grief and strength and paves the way for a future filled with hope.

The Journey of Grief and Closure

Grief is a complex journey, a profound and often solitary path that touches the deepest parts of your Spirit. It is a natural response to loss and a testament to our shared love and connection. While the pain of loss can be overwhelming, sacred ceremonies offer a beacon of hope and a pathway to healing. They provide structure, meaning, and a sense of continuity, helping us navigate the tumultuous seas of grief and move towards acceptance, peace and closure.

Closure is not a brunt end but a metamorphosis. It is the gentle unfolding of acceptance, the softening of sharp edges. Through ceremony, a bereaved mother navigates the labyrinth of her grief, finding moments of clarity and peace. She acknowledges the pain, celebrates the joy and releases the weight of guilt, emerging with a heart that, though scarred, beats with a deeper wisdom.

The power of sacred ceremony lies in its ability to weave the threads of grief and hope into a fabric that wraps you in bone-deep healing. It is a testament to the resilience of the human spirit, a celebration of the eternal bond between mother and child and a gentle reminder that in the dance of life and death, there is always a place for love to flourish.

Finding Closure Through Ritual

Closure does not mean forgetting. It signifies reaching a place of acceptance and peace with the courage to keep living and loving. Sacred ceremonies can facilitate this process by allowing mothers to:

- **Acknowledge the Pain:** Recognising and validating grief as the first step towards healing. Rituals provide a safe space to confront and express their pain.
- **Celebrate Life:** Remembering the joy and love the child brought into their lives helps balance the sorrow with gratitude.
- **Release Guilt and Regret:** Mothers can let go of any lingering guilt or regret through acts of forgiveness and self-

compassion, understanding that their love was always enough.
- **Reconnect with Themselves**: Grief can make mothers feel disconnected from their identity. Sacred ceremonies offer a path back to self-awareness and self-care.

Rituals of Remembrance

- **Lighting a Candle:** The simple act of lighting a candle can symbolise the enduring light of the child's spirit. Each flicker of the flame serves as a reminder that their love and memory continue to illuminate the mother's heart.
- **Writing Letters:** Composing letters allows the Mother to express her deepest emotions, regrets, and love. These letters can be kept in a special box, read aloud, or even burned in a release ritual, symbolising letting go of pain and embracing healing.
- **Ritual of Release:** Write down feelings of pain, anger, or grief on small pieces of paper. Burn the papers in a safe container as a symbolic act of releasing the trauma. It won't serve you to continually carry the heaviness of that which you cannot control or change. Release the grip it has on you, Let it go so you can live and create.
- **Planting a Tree or Garden**: Creating a living memorial in a tree or garden can offer a tangible connection to the child. Watching the tree grow or tending to the garden can become meditative, fostering a sense of ongoing connection and life.
- **Flower Ritual:** Gather flowers to use as a vehicle to share your prayers, love and blessings to honour the child's Spirit. Find a body of water that feels sacred and release the flowers into the water, which cleanses your spirit.

Moving Forward with Grace

As time passes, the intensity of grief may lessen, but the memory of the life remains ever-present. Sacred ceremonies can become annual traditions or spontaneous acts of remembrance that continue to honour the child's Spirit. Ultimately, these rituals are not just about mourning; they are about celebrating the profound bond between mother and child, a bond that transcends physical presence and continues to inspire love, strength and resilience. Through sacred ceremonies, bereaved mothers can find a way to navigate their sorrow, embrace their memories and move forward with grace, knowing that their child's spirit is forever a part of their journey.

13

THE LANGUAGE OF BIRTH
NAVIGATING THE INITIATION OF BIRTH AND THE PRIMAL WILD

"The Birthing Woman is the original shaman. She brings the ancestral spirit being into this realm while risking her life doing so. No wonder that the most ancient temples were the sacred birthplaces and that the priestesses of the Mother were also midwives, healers, astrologers and guides to the souls of the dying. Women bridge the borderline realms between life and death and in the past have therefore always been the oracles, sibyls, mediums and wise women"

-Monica Sjöö

Birth is a language. Even though no birth is ever the same, some birth characteristics stand the test of time. Becoming familiar with this language will help you feel empowered. When you know what to expect, you can surrender to it. The female body is an incredible temple of wisdom designed for birth.

In the sacred journey of childbirth, every word spoken carries profound energy, shaping not just the physical experience but also the spiritual and emotional dimensions of the birthing process. Language is key to empowering or disempowering, instilling fear or courage, and shaping the perception of birth as a journey of pain or transformation.

Consider the conventional terminology used in Western medical discourse surrounding childbirth: contractions, delivery, and labour. These words, laden with clinical connotations, often evoke a sense of struggle, pain, and passive endurance. Contractions imply a forceful tightening, a squeezing sensation that can invoke tension and resistance. Delivery suggests a passive reception, as if the birthing Mother is merely a vessel for the baby's arrival. Labour connotes arduous work, a trial to be endured rather than a sacred rite of passage for *the great work* to be birthed through us.

In the realms of spiritual birth, birthing language takes on a different hue that honours the birthing mother's innate wisdom and strength. Words like surges, birthing/borning, and journeying offer a more empowering narrative that aligns with the natural rhythms and cycles of birth. Use these words if they help.

Surges evoke the image of waves, gentle yet powerful movements that ebb and flow, guiding the birthing Mother through each contraction with grace and ease. Instead of holding one's breath in anticipation of pain, they encourage surrender and relaxation, allowing the body to open and expand with each surge.

Birthing, or Borning, embodies the act of bringing forth new life, a sacred dance between the birthing Mother and the baby, guided by intuition and trust. It reframes birth as a collaborative effort, where both Mother and child are active participants in the miracle of creation. Journeying speaks to the transformative nature of childbirth, likening it to a spiritual pilgrimage, a passage of initiation into motherhood or parenthood. It honours the courage, resilience and wisdom required to traverse this sacred threshold.

By reclaiming and reshaping the birth language, we reclaim agency over our birthing experiences, infusing them with intention, reverence and empowerment. Each word becomes a prayer, a mantra that guides us through the sacred portal of birth, reminding us of our inherent strength and divine connection to the miracle of life. That's not to say we cannot use the generally accepted terms like labour, of course we can, it simply means we rise above the energetic imprint these words can have on the psyche. As we honour the spiritual significance of language in birth, we invite the presence of love, peace and grace into the birthing space, allowing for a sacred and transformative experience that transcends the physical realm.

Physiological Birth

Labour and birth typically progress through several physiological stages driven by powerful hormones. Birth is a journey and stages are characterised by specific changes in the cervix, contractions and the baby's descent. In this way, birth is a language and becoming fluent in the physiology of birth will help you become more confident in surrendering to and harnessing your primal power.

THE PRIMARY STAGES of physiological labour and birth are:

1. Early Labour (Latent Phase):

- This stage marks the onset of regular contractions and cervical changes. Contractions are typically mild to moderate in intensity and may be irregular. Cervical dilation begins, usually from 0 to around 3-4 centimetres. The latent phase can last for several hours or even days, especially for first-time Mothers.

2. Active Labour:

- In this stage, contractions/surges become stronger, longer and more regular. Cervical dilation progresses rapidly, usually from around 3-4 centimetres to 7-8 centimetres. The pace of labour quickens and the birthing Mother may feel increased pressure and intensity of contractions. Active labour is often characterised by a sense of focus and determination as the birthing Mother works through each contraction.

3. Transition Phase:

- Transition is the shortest but most intense phase of labour, typically lasting from a few minutes to a couple of hours. It's the point of no return. Contractions reach their peak intensity and frequency, often occurring every 2-3 minutes and lasting around 60-90 seconds. Cervical dilation progresses from around 7-8 centimetres to full dilation (10 centimetres). The birthing Mother may experience intense pressure in the pelvis, rectum and lower back, as well as nausea, shaking and feelings of exhaustion or overwhelm.

4. Second Stage (Pushing Stage):

- This stage begins when the cervix is fully dilated (10 centimetres) and ends with the baby's birth. The birthing mother feels the urge to push as the baby descends through the birth canal. Contractions may become less frequent but more intense, with a strong urge to bear down during each contraction. Generally speaking, the baby's head crowns as it passes through the vaginal opening, followed by the rest of the body. The second stage's duration varies but typically lasts from a few minutes to a couple of hours, depending on factors such as maternal position, baby's position and strength of contractions.

5. Third Stage (Delivery of the Placenta):

- After the baby is born, the uterus continues to contract, expelling the placenta from the uterus. Contractions help to separate the placenta from the uterine wall and push it out through the birth canal. The birthing Mother may experience mild contractions and a sense of fullness as the placenta is delivered. Delivery of the placenta usually occurs within 5-30 minutes after the baby's birth, although it can take longer in some cases.

Each stage of labour and birth is a natural and essential part of the birthing process, guided by the body's innate wisdom and physiology. While the timeline and progression of labour may vary from woman to woman, the language is the same.

The Primal Wild: Understanding the Language of Birth

As you ripen during pregnancy, your energy field expands, slowly stretching dimensions to meet the Spirit of your unborn baby. There is a divine intelligence that exists here and a liminal space where you have all the wisdom of birthing mothers worldwide. This is called the *Birth Field*, and the more sensitive and attuned you are, the easier it is to feel when you start to feel the tendrils of it spiral around you.

The Birth Field

As you begin to activate and enter the *Birth Field*, there may be times when a last flush of doubt and insecurity floods the nervous system. It's as though all the preparation you have been doing start to unravel. This can happen due to relational tension, purging emotions, a seed of fear that someone planted in passing or perhaps your mind simply starts racing with all the what ifs and how you can't do this.

Your mind is a powerful tool that can make or break your birthing experience. Amongst the storm, you must find your centre. This is rooted deeply in the presence of the now, where everything is as it is. In any type of transformational journey work, the key is to come back into the body and the breath. The breath is the life force that courses through your blood; it connects us to the Spiritual dimensions and our bodies.

Using your breath can soothe and calm your adrenaline response, help you manage intense emotional and physical pain and go deeper into *the Great Mystery*. It is beneficial to practice directing your breath through your body before you give birth, as this will give you a reference point from which to work. With long and deep inhalation, you can direct your breath to areas of the body that feel out of alignment, especially your mind and bring everything back into a state of homeostasis.

A fantastic visualisation when feeling off-kilter is to imagine yourself as a strong and mighty tree. Breathe in the visual of this and send roots deep into Mother Earth. The tree trunk is sturdy and strong, grounded deeply into the heart of the Mother, whilst the branches ebb and flow, dancing with the storm. The tree may bend and flex a little, depending on the nature of the storm, though it continues to stand strong, resilient and undisturbed in the truth of its presence.

Trusting Your Primal Body Wisdom

To trust your body's wisdom, you must learn to listen. Trusting your body to open and surrender fully to this incredible initiation will leave you in awe and fill you with incredible strength, power and wisdom you have never experienced.

Birth is a language. When you allow yourself to become familiar with the way your body speaks to you, when you immerse yourself in positive and uplifting birth stories from other women and also permit yourself to switch off and listen, you will enter into the *primal wild,* where all birthing mothers before you, help to sing you and your baby through.

During the later stages of pregnancy, your intuition will become heightened, and your dreaming may be more potent as it helps you process and release any hidden fears. You may begin to anchor in the blueprint of your birthing journey with visions and premonitions. You may begin to have this niggly feeling that something may not be right or that things are shifting. You may have a sudden urge to move your body in a particular way, visit a sacred site, tie up loose ends etc. Trust this.

Trust the way that your body speaks to you. As you cross the threshold into *the Great Mystery*, energy will ripple through your body. You may want to make certain sounds or move in a particular way. In this space, you are activating your primal nature. You may embody different animalistic expressions. You may feel like you are bursting with electricity and primal power. The energy surges will move through you, clearing the channels if you let them. Do not be frightened of this.

When I was in labour with Auraura, my firstborn, I remember being in the bathtub swaying gently; I had left the physical plane and was travelling through psychedelic landscapes of rich colour and texture. A peaceful and serene sense of calm washed through my body and I began to wail. The attending midwife sat in the corner, simply observing. I'll never forget the look on her face when I would come back into my body, she had an expression of such humbled awe. The sounds kept coming and from memory, I began to sing like a whale.

As my baby descended into my pelvis slowly, the sounds pulled me into a deep aquatic realm of grace and beauty. Everything in that moment stood still. It's as if I was floating, totally immersed in the birthing waters of the Divine, carrying my whale song.

Fast forward to the transition stage, and that serenity was replaced with primal roaring, deep guttural moaning, commanding my baby down with each breath. It is important that birthing Mothers feel safe to access these primal states. Most mammals will retreat into a quiet and dark space to give birth. So do women. Most of the time, it is within their own being.

When you surrender to your primal body wisdom, you can feel a subtle movement that brings the baby closer to you. You must get out of your head and into your body. You can't think your way through birth... the only way out is in. Go inwards. Trust and Surrender is the name of the game.

The Drop

As you ripen, you will notice that you can suddenly breathe a little easier. This is because your pregnant belly would have dropped as the baby aligns into a lower position and becomes engaged in the pelvis. You will know when you have dropped because of the shape and if you can place at least 3 finger spans from the top of your ribs to the top of the fundus. Depending on the baby's position, you may notice some "space" at the top, like a squishy feeling. You will also feel like you can take deep breaths again as the pressure is taken off the diaphragm

Braxton Hicks

In 1872, John Braxton Hicks investigated the later stages of pregnancy and noted that many women felt contractions without being near birth. Often called 'false' labour, some women experience this as a natural practice run. Braxton-Hicks contractions are unpredictable, do not occur regularly, and do not become more intense over time. They're more like tightening sensations.

However, they serve the purpose of bringing to the surface any unresolved emotion or tension so that you can clear the way for birth.

Early Labour

Signs of labour include feeling restless, indecisive, moody, very emotional, experiencing lower back and abdominal pain, loose bowel movements and the mucous plug dislodging or membranes 'waters' rupturing.

Most women experience their water breaking as a gush of fluid. It should be clear and mostly odourless or sweet-smelling. If it's yellow, green or brown, contact your medical provider immediately, as this signifies the baby has passed meconium and may be stressed. In post-term babies, it is not uncommon to have stained waters.

Mucous Plug/ Bloody Show

In my 2 earlier pregnancies, I did not experience the mucous plug or water breaking. I had a bloody show at around 6cm dilation in established labour. All of my babies were birthed with bulging forewaters, and the amniotic sac did not break until they were crowning.

With Auruara, my first land birth, I had the midwife rupture the membranes for me to help relieve the pressure, though I am now convinced that if we had left it, she would have been born *en caul,* meaning born with the amniotic sac intact. En Caul births are quite auspicious in that they are rare, with odds at 1 in 80,000.

The mucous plug can be passed and then grow back again, in that it has not fully dislodged and could mean labour is another 2-3 weeks away. With my 3rd baby, I was able to experience a true spontaneous labour I passed my mucous plug 3 days before labour. It was clear and gluey, much like ovulation mucous, but more of it.

The following night, after a beautiful lovemaking session, I remember feeling wet on my inner thighs. When I went to the toilet (as I always do after sex), I noticed that when I wiped, there was a thick creamy mucous.... and lots of it.

After I peed and wiped again, I noticed there was a tinge of blood. This was indeed a bloody show, which meant my cervix was ripe and my body was signalling it was ready and labour was close.

Every birth is different, so don't get too caught up in overthinking if you don't have a show or your waters break. I only experienced my waters gushing with my 4th birth and was quite surprised at how much liquid there was. Thankfully, I was at home, and it happened the morning of his birth.

Prodromal Labour

As early labour begins, you will descend into your body and expand into the cosmos. You may feel your senses heightened and you may become very sensitive to sounds, smells and external stimuli. As labour progresses, you must do what you can to keep calm and keep moving as you would naturally. If you've planned to give birth in a hospital or birthing centre, notify the staff, but do not go until you know you know it is established labour, providing it is safe for you to do so.

Surges will grip you and pull you inwards, into the zone, into the Spiral. They usually start in the lower back and sweep around to the front of your womb, lasting a few seconds and as they progress, they will begin to intensify in sensation and frequency. Usually lasting between 30-60 seconds and 20-5 minutes apart. Your big, beautiful belly will feel tight and you may notice your belly button pointing downwards.

Once the rhythm is established and you know that labour is beginning, it is the best time to light a candle. Let your trusted inner circle know that 'it's time' so that they can light their candles too or do whatever ceremony or prayers to help you sing your baby in. Begin to time your surges. You know you are entering into active labour when they have a regular and consistent rhythm.

Active Labour

Once you have established that you are in labour, it is best to ensure you have everything you need on hand to surrender to your primal body wisdom fully. A general rule is that you are in true labour when you've had surges lasting for a minute, five minutes apart, for an hour. Having said that, you may begin to notice the sequence counting down in minutes, so over the span of an hour, you may go from 20min, 12, 8,7,7,5,5,4,3,2 and by the time the surges are 2mins apart you probably won't be timing anymore!

You may vomit during the surges as they begin to intensify, they may make you feel woozy and disorientated. You must feel safe and secure while you ride the surges. Remember, with each one that washes over you, to allow them to come like waves. Use your breath to navigate through them and focus on the physiological side of birth that you are experiencing in the baby's descent.

Each surge shows you that the baby is being pushed against your cervix, helping it to dilate and open to get ready for birth. The more you allow yourself to feel and surrender and open into the feminine, the easier your birthing experience will be. Breath is the key here, as with any transformational journeywork.

You may feel jittery and anxious, experience hot flushes and feel your nerves on edge. You may have bowel movements or be insatiably hungry or horny. If you are still smiling and chatty, know you have not reached transition yet. Keep moving your body, spiralling your hips and adopt a semi-upright position that is comfortable, to let gravity help do the work.

Transition

Transition is such a majickal stage of labour.

Why do I say this? Well, it is the defining moment that a woman realises they are indeed in the grips of an initiation; there is NO turning back now.

The transition will bring up all your insecurities and trigger your fight-or-flight response. This happens because you are getting shots of adrenaline through your body to help move your bones so the baby can move through your pelvis. Don't be surprised if your confidence wanes during this time. It is important to focus on deep breaths, relaxing your jaw and softening your body during the surge.

You might vocalise or internalise dialogue, like,

"I can't do this, I've had enough now. Give me the drugs, can I have an epidural now, I just want to run away, I seriously can't do this anymore"

The transition will allow you to come up against your edges; it will consume you in the moment's intensity, like a crescendo of sensation, until you break through to the other side. This is the moment where the *Maiden* needs to step aside. She can not walk through this portal- this is the moment where you leave everything you've ever known, every mask and skin you've worn and you unravel into the mystery, completely stripped of your identity to claim your Mother self. The transition has you at the edge of birth's door, peering through and leaning in until your moment comes to step through, crossing the threshold into the unknown. If you are birthing in water, you should get in the bath right on transition, if not just before.

Ride the Surge

Redefining labour pain as intense sensations will allow you to move with them. I prefer to call them surges rather than contractions because they feel like waves crashing at birth's shore. When you ride them, you work with your breath and allow them to wash over you; they may consume you for a moment with a sensory overload, though they will reach a peak and then fall. They can be exhilarating and even orgasmic when you allow yourself to expand with them.

The best thing you can do is the most counterintuitive, soften and relax the moment the surge hits. The easiest way to do this is to focus on relaxing your shoulders, tongue and jaw with long, deep, rhythmic, intentional breathing. This will give you the experience of expanding and opening to receive your child and make the whole process flow smoothly. When you resist, clench, and contract with pain, you take yourself out of the driver's seat and become passive in the whole experience. Remember, you are opening into the cosmos, so open. Breathe, surrender, open and flow.

Birth

After the transition stage, there is this beautiful experience of working with the surges as if they were a wave, you are now on the surfboard riding it to shore. It is probably not as fun, but it is an exhilarating ride!

You will begin to experience the surges intensify. You may feel exhausted, like you can't go on. This is a great stage to have a small spoon of honey or a drink of juice if you can stomach it to keep your blood sugar levels up. Sipping on ice can help to keep you hydrated, especially if you have vomited.

As the pressure in your pelvis builds and the baby begins to make its way through your birth canal, you may have a bowel movement. This is perfectly natural and is nature's way of inoculating beneficial bacteria into the baby's gut to give them a healthy microbiome. Gut health is a hot topic in the health field and there is plenty of research on it. The bacteria present in the vaginal canal go in through the baby's nose and mouth and find their way into the gut. Eating healthy foods and taking probiotics are important so that the baby gets good bacteria.

There is no reason to fear having a bowel movement, no need to be embarrassed as it is quite common. Simply do what you need to do to wipe the area clean if you're having a land birth and if you are water birthing, scoop the poop out of the water. My midwife told me the solution to pollution is dilution!

Keeping your focus inwards and inside your body, you can begin your shamanic journey to collect your child, crossing the rainbow bridge and meeting in the spiritual planes. This usually happens in the peak intensity of the surges as the body stretches, when a sense of calm and stillness washes over you as you are transported out of your body, into the Great Mystery, to meet your newborn, soul to soul. You may have a rush of emotion upon meeting in this place, and it may become a peak Spiritual experience that will continue to shape your life for years to come.

When you are both ready, you cross the threshold and meet at the sacred gate, your cervix. When the cervix is fully dilated, you may have a natural urge to push- this is called 'bearing down', and it puts you back into your seat of power, physically, as you are now completely facilitating this birth with your body and baby.

Stay anchored in your body using your breath and talking to baby; you can journey together to breathe baby through and out. It is ideal to use the power of gravity and seek to be in positions that favour this; kneeling, squatting, and all fours are great empowering ways to give birth. If you take the position of a wide-legged squat, it can help to open up the pelvis by a couple of centimetres, which makes it easier for the baby to come through. This is great to know if the baby feels stuck.

If you are pushing, you want to focus on the muscles you would use to move your bowels, focus on your strength and breathe into deep grunting sounds. In all ways, whether you are vocal or not, you want the sound to move downwards, so use deep guttural sounds that connect to your primal and raw power as a Woman.

As the baby moves through the birth canal, you may feel the 'corkscrew' action. This can feel incredibly unnerving because you are so open and receptive. You may notice no reprieve between surges now. They can come one after the other. Conserve your energy as best you can by breathing deeply and softening into full surrender. Let your body do what it needs to. This is the time for you to surrender deeply to the *primal wild.* It is important to keep talking to the baby and breathing deeply and rhythmically, focusing on relaxing your jaw and throat. Do whatever you can to let go. You're here. It's happening. Your body knows EXACTLY what it needs to do; your job is to facilitate the birth of your baby and yourself as a Mother.

This initiation requires you to yield to the full power of the feminine.

The more you resist, the longer it will take and the harder it will be. The reality and what I know to be true from embodied birth wisdom, is that birth can be an ecstatic, orgasmic and joyful moment of profound spiritual connection and clarity. To reach this space, you will have to deprogram yourself from a couple of hundred years of patriarchal fear-based programming and allow yourself to receive the medicine of a millennium of empowered grandmothers and birth keepers.

So, as the moment of 'crowning' arrives, it is important to be fully present on your throne, in complete Sovereign expression as an empowered birthing Mother. This is the domain where you learn to trust yourself, this is the domain where you adorn yourself with your own power.

Allow yourself to stretch, expand and meet the edges of the universe. You are a sacred portal and your baby is here. As the perineum stretches, it may feel like fire or an intense scorching sting. That is because your vagina, labia and perineum have reached maximum capacity to expand, as the skin is elastic. The more you breathe through this, the more it can stretch and open. Beathe. Breathe through the intense sensations. On the other side of this is your baby.

Birthing the head is the hardest part, so remember this because it won't matter how the baby presents itself. If the baby presents head first, then once the head is out, there will be a moment of relief; the surges will then help the baby release the rest of its body from your vagina.

It is important that if you are in water, you stay low. The outside air that touches the baby's skin triggers a breathing response. If in water, after a small pause, bring the baby to the surface face down so that the water does not go up the nose and cause choking and spluttering. You can suction mucous and fluid out of the baby's nose using your mouth to ensure the airways are clear.

If you have postpartum herbs on standby, take your tinctures under the tongue

The Birth Pause

Some women experience what is known as the birth pause, and in my experience, this happens in two very powerful sequences that can be easy to miss.

The first is when the baby fully descends into the birth canal, usually when crowning. The Mother may instinctually rest, surrendering to her breath as she allows the surges to wash over her whilst she regains strength for the emergence of her child. This pause also gives the perineum time to stretch to full capacity, which will minimise the potential of tearing as she breathes the baby through.

Another pause can also happen immediately after the baby has been born, especially with land births. This pause is a natural response and integration period for both Mother and baby, as the Spirit of each return to the body.

It is important that the Mother is undisturbed and not rushed during this natural integration period as she mentally and emotionally processes the profound opening of her body as she lands back into herself from crossing over into a different dimension to receive her child. When she has gathered herself and is ready, she will reach for her baby, thus consciously claiming her baby and role as Mother. This powerful moment shapes a womans psyche, as she comes to accept the completion of this stage of her initiation, transitioning from *Maiden*, birthing her baby and herself as a *Mother*. The birth of a baby, is also the birth of a Mother.

Becoming the Birth Shaman

The word shaman crosses many different cultures. In the English language, it is derived from the areas of Russia and goes back a few centuries. It relates to a person within a community who can access different spiritual dimensions. Shamans were the so-called seers and mystics, the wisdom and medicine keepers and those who could walk between worlds.

Birth is bigger than the moment. You're not just giving birth to your child. You're giving birth to yourself as a mother and a new timeline that you and your beautiful child will create and walk together in a relationship. A new Spiral. This journey opens up the possibilities for you both to connect with the role of an ancestor. It allows you to connect with something bigger than this physical reality. You are connecting with the pristine origins of humanity. The template of birth and creation.

The template of birthing the world is that we consistently dream into being... dreaming ourselves awake. As a birth shaman, you have an incredible privilege to access these spiritual dimensions to seed your own vision and a bigger dream for all of humanity as a collective. You can connect with your child's soul in one dimension and guide and breathe it through the portal of birth into this dimensional plane. This usually transpires around the stage of transition as the surges sweep you away, through the spiral where you can have out-of-body experiences and DMT like hallucinations.

It is an individual journey for each birthing Mother to connect with all that is. All timelines. All consciousness. You become the sacred bridge. You walk between worlds. You become the seer and medicine woman. As you allow yourself to open and embrace the enigma of life, your birth journey, no matter what happens, will be a medicine walk. In this way, you allow yourself to unhook from the fear or any potential reality not completely aligned with what you need to walk and master in your lifetime.

WISDOM KEEPERS transmute and alchemise the energy of pain into purpose and medicine. Alchemise the deep body sensations to expand into creativity as you birth your baby. Every potential reality is open to you in the primal wilderness of the Birth Field, you can access untapped, pure consciousness.

So when you journey into that space, it is essential to enter with a clear heart and mind and allow *the Great Mystery* to reveal itself to you as you reach out and collect your child from the spiritual worlds, crossing the rainbow bridge. You can explore the landscape of this holographic dimension, it may feel like a lifetime has passed in a few seconds. Receive the medicine of the primal wild, create a map and bring it back to share with others.

Women are the wisdom keepers of the womb and can radically transform this paradigm and revolutionise how we experience the imprints of love and truth. Embodying the birthkeeper and claiming those roles so we can walk them deeply connected to Spirit and Nature helps us restore the sacred codes of birth. Peace on earth begins with birth, and you must recognise that you have the power to imprint yourself as a Mother and your child so that you have a connection to heart, spirit and place.

I encourage you to sit with the possibility of what you could access in this primal space, *The Great Mystery*. This dimension is ONLY available to birthing mothers, and only the initiates with clear eyes to see will receive the vast wisdom of the women's mysteries. Embodying the birth shaman allows you to walk between worlds in an empowering way.

Birth in its own rite is completely transformational and entering this space with this wisdom is a complete game changer, especially if you have a sacred mission as a visionary who is here to change the world radically. If you feel the calling deep in your bones that there is a different way for us to all experience this world more holistically and peacefully, then I encourage you to sit with this concept and invitation to become the *Birth Shaman*, because those with a big vision and pure intention can harness the energy of the birth field to empower their bigger dreaming for a brighter, symbiotic future for all generations.

The ripple effects that come from birth by a mother rooted in her power are profound. This force is moving through timelines and blood, activating the cellular memory of this ancient wisdom and is why women are feeling this calling to remember the sacred birthing ways and to connect more deeply with birth as an initiation and *sacred rite of passage* so that our babies are energetically attuned to a new way of being.

There is medicine around each birth that will reveal a depth of yourself that you may not have acknowledged before. Tuning into your womb will allow you to be open to receiving yourself more fully and commit to your innate power and truth of what it is you are here to do and birth in service to the greater good of all.

WHEN I WAS FIRST INITIATED into this realm, it completely transformed my world and showed me all of the ways I was out of alignment with my truth and purpose for being of service in this space and time. It brought death to the old and helped me birth the most authentic embodiment of my soul's calling. I knew I was here to be more, that my magnum opus was beyond the legacy I was creating as a Mother. It became clear that I had a lot of work to do in this world. Lead by Spirit, I knew that my purpose work was connected to a bigger dreaming...One that equally excited and terrified me.

14

PRACTICAL BIRTHING WISDOM
REMEMBER TO BREATHE AND RELAX YOUR JAW!

> "We must attempt to tell the whole truth about birth, the truth that includes the transformation, mastery, satisfaction, personal power and the difference between pain and suffering."
> – Cheri van Hoover

When I became pregnant for the first time, I immersed myself in research about birth. I wanted to know everything; what to expect, potential complications, emergency procedures, and more. As a critical overthinker, this knowledge helped to quiet my mind. I understood that birth was a sacred initiation, one that would stretch me in ways I couldn't fully comprehend beforehand.

In the season of the *Maiden*, everything is new and unknown. The profound experience of birth is something you cannot truly fathom until you are in the midst of it. No matter how much research you do, you will never be fully ready because you are not meant to be. You learn by doing, being present in the moment and by allowing the energy of birth to guide you. In this way, the emerging Mother in you becomes a sacred bridge, a conduit for the divine, for Spirit to move through you. Birth is an initiation into your power and trusting your journey as a Mother. It is the ultimate act of sacred service.

It is crucial to understand the stages of transformation your body undergoes and the language of birth, as discussed in the previous chapters. This knowledge helps you stay present and centred in your power as you navigate the great mystery of birth. It provides you with a map and a sense of direction so that you can trust in your initiation as you traverse the *primal wild*. When you become fluent in this language, understand the processes at play and trust the journey as an initiation into a new reality and state of being, it becomes easier to surrender and become deeply embodied in your experience.

Understanding the Hormonal Journey and the Importance of an Undisturbed Environment

The physiology of birth is a beautifully orchestrated symphony of hormonal fluctuations and physiological changes designed to facilitate the safe and successful passage of new life into the world. Understanding the hormonal journey underscores the importance of creating an undisturbed environment that supports the natural progression of labour. By honouring the body's innate wisdom and providing a safe, supportive atmosphere, you can optimise hormonal balance, promote relaxation and embrace the transformative journey of childbirth with confidence and grace.

Throughout labour and childbirth, a woman's body undergoes a remarkable series of hormonal shifts orchestrated by the intricate interplay of various hormones. Oxytocin, often referred to as the love hormone or hormone of labour, plays a central role in initiating and sustaining contractions. Released in response to physical touch, intimacy and emotional support, oxytocin promotes the rhythmic uterine contractions necessary for labour's progression. Endorphins, the body's natural pain-relieving hormones, are also released during labour, helping to mitigate discomfort and promote relaxation. Additionally, adrenaline levels may increase slightly during the early stages of labour, providing an extra surge of energy and focus, especially during the transition when the pelvis opens in preparation for the baby to enter the birth canal.

Creating an undisturbed environment is paramount for facilitating the natural progression of labour and optimising hormonal balance.

Distractions, interruptions and unnecessary interventions can disrupt the delicate hormonal dance of birth, potentially hindering smooth progression and stalling labour. In an undisturbed environment, a woman feels safe, secure and supported, allowing her body to release oxytocin freely and enter a state of deep relaxation conducive to labour. This sense of safety and privacy is essential for promoting the release of endorphins, which help manage pain and enhance the birthing experience. By minimising external stimuli and providing continuous emotional and physical support, caregivers can foster trust and confidence, empowering women to navigate the birth journey with strength and confidence.

In an undisturbed environment, you can surrender to the great mystery of birth, allowing yourself to be vulnerable and tapping into your inherent strength and resilience. You can welcome your baby into the world with love, joy and empowerment. Creating such an environment allows the body to navigate through each stage of birth instinctively with minimal intervention.

The Power of Breath and Relaxation

Fear releases cortisol and adrenaline, inhibiting labour by counteracting the calming effects of oxytocin and endorphins. Deep conscious breathing stimulates the parasympathetic nervous system, which decreases heart rate and blood pressure, fostering a sense of calm and relaxation. This practice helps manage pain and maintain focus during labour.

Ina May Gaskin's *Sphincter Law* teaches us that the cervix, like other sphincters in the body, functions best when a woman feels safe and unobserved. This underscores the importance of a calm, supportive environment where a woman can feel relaxed and undisturbed.

Intentionally using your breath to flow with the surges as they come, using deep, rhythmic breathing through the sensations will help you expand beyond the contractions and open the floodgates of endorphins to work their majick. You must be present with this process and try not to hold your breath during the intense sensations. Trying to resist or control your way through labour surges will create more body tension and is counterproductive towards a blissful birth, which requires your surrender. When you feel the contraction, you need to use your breath to expand around it. Use your breath to exhale the tension, each time relaxing your shoulders and your jaw, softening into the rhythm of the surges and reaching a crescendo, where you breathe your baby through.

The Womb-Throat Connection

The throat and the womb share a fascinating connection that dates back to embryonic development. The neck is called the cervical spine, and the lower portion of the uterus is called the cervix. During the embryonic stage, these structures grow together before they separate as the fetus develops. This connection persists, linking the throat and the pelvic floor through fascial tissue.

The vagus nerve, the longest and most complex of the 12 cranial nerves, plays a crucial role in this connection. It contributes to the autonomic nervous system (ANS), regulating involuntary physiological processes such as heart rate, respiration, digestion and sexual arousal. The vagus nerve has three distinct divisions: the *sympathetic*, which manages the threat response of fight/flight; the *parasympathetic*, which manages rest and digestion; and the *enteric*, which manages gastrointestinal functions.

The larynx and cervix are connected via the vagus nerve and the jaw and pelvis are linked through a web of connective tissue called fascia. Our mouth, jaw and womb develop from the same membrane in utero. This shared origin explains why they not only look similar but are also functionally interconnected. The relaxation of the mouth and jaw can facilitate the relaxation of the pelvic floor, aiding the birthing process. So, if you must engage the mind during birth, remember to focus on **relaxing your jaw**.

The Role of Movement in Childbirth

Movement in childbirth is a vital element that aligns with the natural rhythms and needs of the labouring body. Throughout labour, a woman's instinctual movements like walking, swaying, squatting, or even simply changing positions can facilitate the progress of labour and provide immense comfort. Each movement helps harness the power of gravity, aiding the baby's descent through the birth canal and ensuring optimal positioning. This dynamic interaction with one's environment promotes the physical progression of labour. It empowers the birthing woman to harness the energy in the *birth field* and engage actively in her birthing process, enhancing her sense of control and agency.

Moreover, movement in childbirth serves as a profound communication between the body and the baby, a dance of mutual cooperation. Upright positions such as standing or squatting can open the pelvis, creating more space for the baby to navigate. Gentle rocking, hip circles or using a birthing ball can alleviate pain and reduce the need for medical interventions. Encouraging freedom of movement allows the labouring woman to respond intuitively to her body's cues, fostering a connection to her innate wisdom and strength. This freedom transforms the birthing environment into a sanctuary of trust and surrender, where the mother can fully embody the powerful journey from *Maiden to Mother*.

The Reawakening: Birth as a Catalyst for Remembering Power and Vitality

In the sacred dance of birth, a woman reconnects with the deepest layers of her being, rediscovering a power and vitality that have always resided within her. As contractions surge like the rhythmic waves of the ocean, she is reminded of her primal essence, the ancient strength that pulses through her veins. Each breath and movement becomes a testament to her resilience and tenacity, a celebration of life itself.

As she traverses the thresholds of pain and transcendence, she awakens to creation's raw, unfiltered energy. The barriers between her mind and body dissolve, leaving her attuned to the wisdom that flows from within. In this crucible of transformation, she is both vulnerable and invincible, cradled by the timeless dance of life and death, contraction and expansions.

The intense journey reveals to her the magnificent capacity of her body, a vessel designed not only to nurture and sustain but to bring forth new life. In this profound initiation, she glimpses the divine spark within herself, the same spark that ignited the stars and breathed life into the universe.

In this moment of sacred birth, she becomes a conduit for the divine, a living embodiment of the creative force that courses through all things. She is reborn alongside her child, emerging from the experience with a renewed sense of purpose and a profound recognition of her inherent power. This realisation imprints itself upon her soul, a reminder that she is a vibrant, powerful being capable of extraordinary feats. The memory of this journey stays with her as she carries it forward into her life as a mother.

The Transformative Power of Birth

Birth is not just a physical act but a profound spiritual awakening. As a woman navigates the labyrinth of labour, she encounters the raw, untamed forces within herself. Often, dormant forces surge to the forefront, illuminating her path with newfound clarity and strength. In the throes of labour, she learns to trust her body's wisdom, to surrender to the primal rhythms that guide her. This trust fosters an unshakeable confidence, not just in her ability to birth but in her capacity to face and overcome life's challenges.

In the stillness between contractions, a deep introspection occurs. In these quiet moments, she connects with generations of women who have birthed before her, drawing strength from the collective experience of womanhood. This connection to the ancestral lineage of mothers grounds her, making her feel supported and never alone. She becomes acutely aware of the cyclical nature of life, understanding that she is part of a continuum, a sacred thread woven into the fabric of existence.

Emerging from the transformative experience of birth, a woman carries a sense of accomplishment and empowerment. She has faced the intensity of creation and has come out the other side not just as a Mother but as a warrior, a creator, and a vessel of life. This transformation instils a deeper appreciation for her body and its incredible capabilities. It redefines her perception of pain, seeing it now as a vehicle for growth and transformation rather than mere suffering.

The journey of birth ignites a fierce love and protectiveness for her child, a bond forged through shared experience. This bond is a testament to her strength and resilience, a reminder of the power that lies within her. She steps into her new role with a renewed sense of purpose, knowing she has been entrusted with nurturing and guiding a new life.

In all its raw beauty and intensity, birth is a powerful reminder of a woman's aliveness. It strips away the superficial, revealing the core of her being, a radiant, powerful and resilient soul. In embracing this experience fully, she reclaims her divine feminine power, awakening to the limitless possibilities within her.

She stands as a Mother and a living embodiment of life's potential, ready to embrace the future with an open heart and unwavering strength. To transform oneself is to transform all of existence.

Through the act of birth, she becomes the architect of the future. With each child she births, she expands herself and the universe.

PART IV- SACRED POSTPARTUM
CROSSING THE THRESHOLD OF MAIDEN TO MOTHER

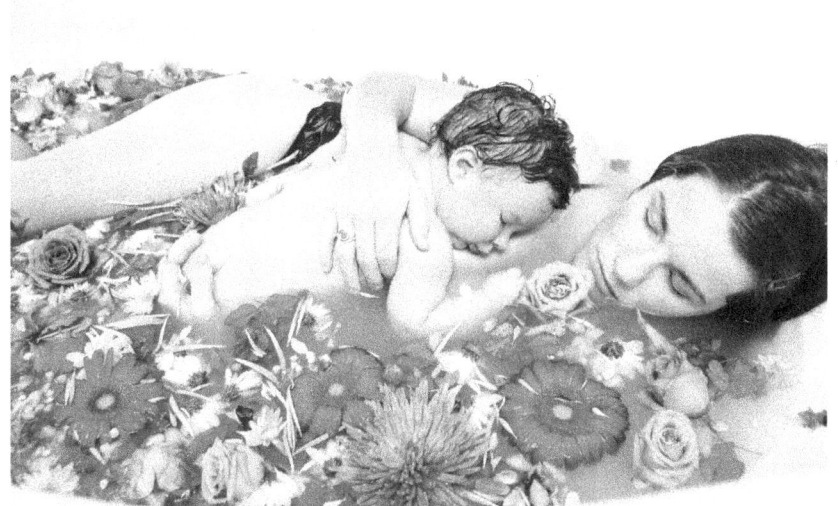

"Sometimes when you pick up your child you can feel the map of your own bones beneath your hands, or smell the scent of your skin in the nape of his neck. This is the most extraordinary thing about motherhood - finding a piece of yourself separate and apart that all the same you could not live without."- Jodi Picoult

15

MOTHER

A NEW WORLD IS BORN

Giving birth is a transformation and it doesn't matter whether you've had eight babies before. It's still a transformation the next time you have another baby, because you are no longer the same woman you were before you had that baby."
– Penny Handford

The process of becoming a mother is called Matresence. It relates to the physical, psychological, emotional and spiritual changes you go through after the birth of your child. It is the journey of becoming a mother and deepening into your role as a matriarch and living ancestor.

Becoming a mother is incredibly powerful. It is '*The Great Work*' in the sense that your role is to not only grow another human being inside your body and nurture that child into maturity, you are also responsible for shaping another being's consciousness and their way of experiencing the world, their formal imprints and how they experience love, feel safe in their body and share their life force and creativity with the world.

Keeping all of this in mind- you are also teaching this new being how to relate by modelling behaviours and regulating sensory input. If unprepared it can feel like a lot of pressure. The journey ahead can short-circuit and overwhelm the nervous system, inviting fear, insecurity and doubt. You have to remember that you not only birthed a baby, you are birthing yourself and this will take time to integrate as you get to know yourself in your new body, role and perspective.

New Identity

Permit yourself to linger in the *Mystery* for as long as needed. You don't have to have it all figured out because you won't! Meet yourself where you are as a woman who has just navigated birth's initiation. Everything following the completion of physiological birth will still be revealed to you moment to moment as you gently cross the threshold from *Maiden to Mother*. You have arrived. Acknowledge that you are here now.

Writing down your thoughts and feelings during this time will help you to process the birth and your transition into your new identity. You may even like to use this time to record your birth story whilst it's fresh in your heart and mind.

It is important to create a safe space to grieve the old life you had, your maidenhood and any fears and insecurities that surface once your baby is earthside. From a spiritual perspective, your Soul has just undergone a massive initiation. As such, you need to prioritise integration time for your Spirit to land back in your body, for your psyche to embrace this identity that is forming and for your nervous system to calm and anchor into this new state of being.

This journey of integration is to be met with tenderness. You have stretched yourself beyond the familiar, so you must give yourself time to understand the language of this new landscape, the shifting hormones and of course, learn the new rhythm of life with your baby.

Bonding

Once your baby is born, you will be in a sacred time of imprinting and bonding. It is important to be as undisturbed as possible. Directly after birth, bringing your baby to your chest will allow them to initiate the *birth crawl*, which is an instinct that will see the baby make its way to your breast. You will be amazed by how strong newborns are, so don't be surprised if they lift their heads and look around the room. Helping your baby latch to your breast will allow the necessary signals to take place that tell your body that your birth is complete.

Oxytocin will help to expel the placenta and elicit the maternal bond. You will have a few minor surges and be able to birth it easily, providing there are no other complications and you remain present in your state of surrender. There is a sense of euphoria once the birth is complete.

You will be awash with hormones and may feel like a Superwoman. Despite feeling like you could run a marathon, it is important to rest and bond. This will create a beautiful starting point for you to claim your role as Mother fully and to set the space to nurture your maternal instincts. Some mothers will feel this immediately; for others, it may take some time to kick into gear. Don't worry if you don't feel bonded immediately; simply be present with what is; you've just birthed your baby and yourself as a new mother. These things can take time, so take the time!

After an hour or so, perhaps once the baby has been checked over and swaddled, it is important to take care of your own needs, like having a warm shower and checking in with your body. Your first visit to the toilet might be an unnerving experience as you still feel quite open. Check for any tears or signs of pelvic organ prolapse. If you do, lean forward to urinate and try the splinting technique to help with bowel movement, whereby you bundle some toilet paper and then use your hand to add pressure to your perineum, covering your vagina. If you are in the hospital, the perfect time to do all this self-care is when the baby is checked for their neo-natal reflexes and APGAR test. Dress yourself in comfortable clothing, and make sure to keep warm.

Coming Home: The Importance of Undisturbed Integration

The most important thing that you can do after giving birth is to rest and nurture yourself and your baby. Your job now is to restore and replenish your body, which has just undergone a mammoth, multi-dimensional initiation and transition from *Maiden to Mother*. Take a moment to fully acknowledge this, and debrief from your birth if you need to. You may still feel energetically open for some time, so be gentle. It is vital to stay warm in the coming weeks and call upon your support network so that you can come back to your centre. Spend some time outside if you can.

Imagine you are a traveller who has just come home after an intense life-changing soul journey and your whole world has been flipped upside down; nothing is quite the same, everything feels different, and all of a sudden, a baby, with no instruction manual, is placed in your hands. What do you do now?

JUST BREATHE, MAMA.

I loved walking barefoot in my garden in the late afternoon sun, feeling the flux of life, with my newborn nuzzled into my chest. A wildly majickal sensation followed me everywhere, a liminal field as I felt my Spirit was still in the other world and I was slowly returning. I felt ecstatic and joyous yet anchored in a deep state of stillness. Everything was pulsing with life, and everything had meaning. A pure state of grace.

Motherhood is more of a marathon than a sprint. It calls you to slow down and surrender to the journey as it unfolds in the moment. You have to be gentle with yourself. This is a time of grace. Give yourself time to integrate, return to your body's presence and get to know your new little soul mate. Allow the first few weeks to be about bonding, sacred imprinting and getting to know your baby and your new mama's body, particularly if breastfeeding.

You do not have to go anywhere if you don't want to. If your environment does not support this deep resting time, see if you can call upon support around you to help lift the load. The idea is to have as much time with minimal pressure to do anything other than rest and be with your baby, though this is not the case for every mother, it is something we must support as a global community. So, if you're reading this and have someone in your community at this stage, perhaps send a friendly message to see if you can help this new mother integrate. It is one of the most beautiful gifts we can give to help create and restore the village around new mothers, especially if a woman is isolated or on her own.

Womb Care

After you feel like you have integrated the energy of birth, you may like to begin your womb care rituals and *'closing of the bones'*, which you'll find in the Womb Healing Section of this book. Spending some time supporting your womb, tending to your blood and staying warm and hydrated is important. It's possible to feel waves of grief pass through your body as you place your hands over your womb. You may miss the sensations of your baby inside of your body, or you may even feel relief that it's all over. You've been on a massive transformative journey, so allow yourself to flow with the emotions as they move through you, witnessing all the sensations.

Energetically connecting with your womb after you've birthed, no matter the outcome, helps you to maintain a strong connection with your body and return home to yourself as a woman and new Mother. It also offers you the space to honour your fertility and your feminine power as a birthing woman.

Sacred Imprinting

In the first few weeks after the baby is born, protecting and guarding the home space is crucial. Despite the stories you hear about many women popping out a baby and then going back to work, if you are privileged enough to be able to rest, then please take it seriously.

During the last trimester, your baby was imprinting on your voice and scent. When babies are born, their sight range is around 20-30cm and quite blurry. They receive sensory information in tones of light and shape. Your areolas get larger and darker because they become a 'target' for the newborn to be able to see and know where food is.

Newborns take in sensory information to help shape their understanding of the world. The visual language is very important. In the waking moments, you may notice your newborn's eyes tracking or darting back and forth, side to side. What they are doing is imprinting important markers on your face and the faces of those close to them. This incredible built-in intelligence allows the baby to create a sense of familiarity and know who is important, who they can trust, and who is kin. It also helps to build healthy oxytocin receptors.

This is why it is so important to protect this space fiercely. Not everyone gets access to you and your newborn immediately. It does not matter how well-meaning friends and extended family are; they don't need to visit or hold your baby if they are not significant to your family. This can sound quite harsh, but the neural pathways your baby creates during this time set them up for life. A newborn's brain has nearly one hundred billion neurons and reaches over half its adult size in the first three months.

The experiences in the first few weeks of life help to program the new baby to healthy love and comfort. Remember the power of *Limbic Imprinting*? It is important to keep your baby close to you, held and safe by Mother's familiar touch and smell. You are the world for your baby.

Attachment

The quality of attachment and care between Mother and child will determine the long-term emotional development of the child. Through sensory stimuli, cognitive and emotional development occurs in the brain and influences how the child will experience relationships with others in the future.

Cultivating a secure attachment bond depends mostly on nonverbal communication between you and your baby. You allow your baby to feel safe and secure when you are present enough to respond to your baby's cues, gestures, sounds, movements and emotional state. That is why it is important to take time to bond with and get to know your baby, keeping them close. Your baby is developing its nervous system and how it responds to this new outside world.

A secure attachment teaches your baby to trust; it will give them the best foundations for life to become a fully realised, empathic, trusting and compassionate adult capable of healthy and intimate relationships with mutual love and respect. This will require your attention and presence.

Trusting and attuning your Maternal Instincts

Your intuition as a mother offers unique insights into your child's needs, emotions and cues, fostering a deep and meaningful connection between you and your child. By trusting your instincts, you can tailor your parenting approach to honour your child's uniqueness, fostering individualised care that promotes their growth and development. This intuitive connection also cultivates a sense of confidence and self-assurance in your role as a mother, empowering you to navigate the uncertainties of parenting with resilience and grace. Trusting your instincts strengthens your bond with your child and fosters self-discovery, revealing your strengths, values and inner wisdom as a Mother. By modelling the importance of intuition and self-trust, you create a supportive environment where your child learns to trust themselves, empowering them to navigate life's challenges confidently and resiliently. In essence, trusting and attuning to your maternal instincts is a transformative practice that honours every mother's innate wisdom, enriching motherhood's journey with depth, authenticity and grace.

Listen to your baby

There is often a misconception that babies are unintelligent, helpless little beings. Whilst they may be incredibly dependent, they are by no means unintelligent. As modern parents, with a bombardment and overload of sensory information, it is imperative that you prioritise learning to listen to your baby and their natural cues in communication.

When I first became a mother, I quickly caught on to Auraura's sounds and body language. She had a 'poo face', which would see her face go bright red, accompanied by little grunts. When she would urinate, she would stop what she was doing as if to concentrate on the sensations of what was happening in her body. She would often get a greyish-blue tinge around her mouth, which would signify that she was holding tension in her belly. Unfortunately, she suffered from intense colic, so she was often screaming. In the early days, I kept feeding her, not knowing if she was screaming because she was hungry or in pain. I felt like a failure.

This led me to observe her intently, and with the help of my mother, who had raised four children, I began to trust that she was well-fed and that her cries were telling me something else. Wind. So I needed to spend more time on making sure she had burped properly before feeding and I would have to allow my milk to flow before putting her to my breast as I had a strong let-down response, which resulted in her half gulping, half choking and swallowing air. After 4 months, I found my groove.

It takes time for you and your baby to learn from each other. Your presence as a mother will help to build a relationship built on connection, and you'll soon be fluent in your baby's cues and natural rhythms, which over time build upon that maternal instinct that will tell you when something is out of the norm. As with learning any language, it simply takes time and practice.

Auraura was toilet trained before she could walk because I knew her body rhythm and cues. This was before I knew *'Elimination Communication'*[1] was a thing!

I remember watching a video in 2007 where Australian mother Priscilla Dunstan[2] shared her discovery of 5 universal sounds babies make during their 'pre-cry' stage. I wish I had known these earlier, but I was thankful that I figured most of them out on my own, and whilst Dunstan allowed this wisdom to go mainstream, I am sure our ancestors knew this.

The 5 universal key sound cues[3] are:

1. Neh: Hunger
2. Eh: Upper wind (burp)
3. Eairh: Lower wind (gas)
4. Heh: Discomfort (hot, cold, wet)
5. Owh/Oah: Sleepiness

There are also movement cues to look out for as well which include;

- Rubbing face: Means baby is tired
- Head rotation: Without crying can mean that your baby is trying to fall asleep and crying can signify discomfort or pain.

- Clenching Fist: Usually means your baby is hungry.
- Arching Back: Usually signifies pain and discomfort with digestion.

Baby Blues

A woman's body undergoes hormonal changes and emotional adjustments during the first few weeks after childbirth. These changes can cause her to feel sad, weepy, irritable, anxious or overwhelmed. It's very common and affects many new mothers, often due to factors like hormonal fluctuations, lack of sleep, physical discomfort and the significant life changes that come with having a new baby.

Physiologically, hormonal shifts play a big role. Pregnancy hormones like estrogen and progesterone drop rapidly after childbirth, which can affect mood. Additionally, there's an increase in stress hormones like cortisol, which can make emotions feel more intense. Sleep deprivation, common in the early postpartum period, can also contribute to feeling more emotional and sensitive.

The 'baby blues' are generally mild and tend to improve independently within a few weeks. However, if feelings of sadness, anxiety or overwhelm persist or worsen, it's important for the new mother to seek support from her healthcare provider, as it could be a sign of postpartum depression, which is a more serious condition that requires treatment.

One of the best things I did was to stay in bed and cry. There was a deep grief that would pass through my body, an innate and primal knowing that an old life or version of me had died. I had to be present with that grief, that pain of growth that cracks your heart wide open so that I could receive the wisdom of surrender.

The Neurodivergent Mother

Neurodivergent mothers face unique challenges in managing sensory overwhelm while caring for an infant during the first few years of life. To support yourself through this period, it's essential to create a sensory-friendly environment at home by minimising clutter and incorporating calming elements like ambient lighting.

Set up functional spaces, like a breastfeeding area stocked with burping towels, water and snacks or a portable nappy changing station. Create these functional spaces in areas you would naturally gravitate towards, rather than pressuring yourself to conform to a new routine. You can optimise these spaces to mitigate stress by anticipating your sensory sensitivities and needs.

Establishing predictable routines for feeding, napping and playtime can provide structure and predictability, helping you to navigate sensory input more effectively. Taking breaks and practicing self-care activities such as deep breathing exercises or short walks outside can help alleviate sensory overload. Additionally, sensory tools like weighted blankets, fidget devices, aromatherapy and soothing music or seeking therapeutic support from professionals specialising in neurodiversity can provide further assistance.

Communicating your needs and boundaries to partners, family and caregivers is crucial, as is practising self-compassion and gratitude amidst parenting challenges. Connecting with other neurodivergent mothers can be incredibly validating and empowering. Through shared experiences, you can gain insights, tips and emotional support to make a difference on your journey and make you feel less alone.

Make no mistake, there will be days when it will feel like absolute chaos. You may feel overstimulated and touched out. You will flip your lid. This is a normal response to sensory overwhelm as it can be a tough gig trying to regulate yourself with the constant demands of raising a child, even more so if they have special needs. In those moments of 'crazy', it is important to remember that you are doing the best you can in a complex situation as a human being with a dysregulated nervous system. Perfection is not the goal.

Some days will feel more like you're surviving rather than thriving, though with time, you will learn how to soothe and regulate your nervous system effectively. Be gentle with yourself and celebrate small victories along the way.

Exploring Intimacy and Sexuality in Motherhood

Contrary to popular belief, the arrival of a child doesn't diminish sensuality; rather, it amplifies it, inviting a deeper exploration of intimacy and desire within the context of sexual expression and eros.

The journey of motherhood brings with it a myriad of physical and emotional changes that can impact the dynamics of intimacy between partners. Sleepless nights, hormonal shifts and the demands of caring for a newborn may initially pose challenges to maintaining a vibrant sexual connection. However, amidst these challenges lies an opportunity, a chance to reignite the flame of passion, connect with new desires and rediscover the erotic connection between lovers.

Open communication is key to nurturing intimacy in the wake of parenthood. Honest conversations about desires, fears, body insecurities and partner expectations create a safe space for lovers to express needs and desires openly. Vulnerability becomes a bridge connecting hearts, allowing partners to deepen their emotional bond as parents and individuals, cultivating a more profound sense of intimacy as a team.

The willingness to embrace change is essential in navigating motherhood's evolving landscape of intimacy. As routines shift and priorities realign, flexibility becomes paramount. So does having a sense of humour. Find creative and playful ways to carve out time for physical intimacy amidst the chaos of parenthood, whether it's stealing a quiet moment during naptime or scheduling regular date nights, engaging in steamy shower play, sensual massages or quickies. Activating and expressing your erotic energy can help to deepen your connectedness with a lover, your body and refine your identity as a sensual woman and Mother. It is ok for you to feel sexy and wanted and to give and receive pleasure.

The Beauty of Being in the Eternal Now

The newborn stage goes by so fast; it may not seem that way when you are in it, but you will be surprised by how quickly your baby grows and changes. The first year of life is where the most transformation occurs, not only for the baby but for you as a new mother.

When you enter the timeless space of the *Now*, it allows you to be in the beauty of being rather than doing. Immerse yourself in the experience of motherhood, when everything is fresh and you and the baby are learning about each other for the first time. Be gentle with yourself and your body. You don't need to be in a hurry to become someone, you already are. Remember, you are the world to your baby.

There is no rush to return to 'normal' life or your 'pre-baby' body. There is a new normal expressing itself daily. From this moment, you get to decide what works for you and your family without any added pressure of trying to make your life a performance akin to a Hollywood movie.

Life is a beautiful mess. You will gradually lose parts of yourself. Let them go for now and surrender to this process as a new power wants to emerge through you. You can be a beautifully messy human who is still completely lovable and capable.

Rest when your baby rests if you feel called to. Slow down and savour every moment, every sniffle, hiccup, cough… every little gesture your baby shares with you. Savour the feeling of the unknown, the newness of it all. Things will shift quickly, so consciously create your memories. This is your life and it's meant for living. Document this sacred time. You will never get it back. Once it's gone, it's gone forever, stored as memory.

In the grand scheme of things, your child is only with you briefly, so show up for life as it is now, in its beautiful mess and confusion, the rawness of this human experience. Be present with the life you choose to live and create daily. This is your path to walk annd your story to write.

Be here, now. There is no other place you need to be.

16

ROOTED IN WISDOM
EMBRACING INDIGENOUS TRADITIONS

"When we respect our blood ancestors
and our spiritual ancestors, we feel rooted."
- Thich Nhat Hanh

Before we walk forward, we must first honour and acknowledge those who have walked before us, not as relics of the past but as living expressions of ancestral wisdom, cultural continuity, resilience and empowerment.

The postpartum experience, universally revered as a sacred and transformative period, finds its depth and richness amplified through the lens of indigenous wisdom. Across cultures and continents, Indigenous communities have cultivated intricate rituals and traditions that honour the birthing couple and their newborn, providing a tapestry of support woven from centuries of human knowledge and spiritual connection.

At the heart of ancient postpartum practices lies a profound reverence for the interconnectedness of life and the natural world, reflecting a deep understanding of humanity's place within this grand web of existence, intertwining the physical, emotional and spiritual realms. These practices serve not only to nurture the physical well-being of mothers and babies but also to foster a sense of belonging, rootedness and community support.

These postpartum traditions offer a poignant reminder of the importance of cultural continuity and resilience. Despite centuries of colonisation, displacement and cultural erasure, Indigenous communities have persisted in safeguarding their traditional knowledge and customs, passing them down through generations as a beacon of resilience and cultural pride. In acknowledging, reclaiming and revitalising these ancestral practices, Indigenous peoples reclaim their agency, identity and sovereignty, forging pathways to healing, empowerment and self-determination.

There are myriad ancient cultural traditions globally that share similarities in practice and reverence of birth as a *sacred rite of passage*.

Sacred Rituals and Practices

Australian Aboriginal communities have their own birthing traditions, which often involve birthing on *country* (ancestral lands) and participating in ceremonies to welcome the newborn and offer blessings for their future. Cultural birthing sites are typically marked by significant landmarks like birthing trees or caves, providing natural settings for labour. Referred to as *"Borning"* in Aboriginal English, these practices are distinct from Western birthing methods and vary between different language groups or Nations, for which there are over 500, each with their own customary laws.

Birth is Women's business and women play central roles in *borning*, with knowledge and rituals passed down through generations, reflecting spiritual and healing approaches rooted in *the Dreaming*, Lore, land, kinship and traditional beliefs about life cycles.

Grandmothers and aunties serve as midwives and birth-keepers, providing practical and spiritual support during childbirth and postpartum, including preparing tools, keeping the fire warm, offering moral support and conducting ceremonies such as song, dance and smoking rituals.

Just before or during birth, the child is given totems, which establish a direct connection to *the Dreaming* and all living beings and land. Other totems are assigned based on the parents' language group, kinship ties and area of belonging, with Aboriginal people holding unique responsibilities to safeguard their totems and ensure their survival. Children received a *'Skin Name'*, directly connected to their ancestral bloodlines and kin group, which were important for determining who they could marry within a *Moitey* system.*

One common postpartum tradition involves burying the placenta, which symbolises diverse beliefs ranging from protecting men from its perceived dangers to serving as a soul map and anchor for the child during future rites of passage.

IN XHOSA CULTURE, childbirth is a communal affair steeped in tradition. Initially, the birth is assisted by grandmothers in a round thatched hut called a rondavel. After giving birth, mothers undergo a period of seclusion lasting around ten days or until the umbilical cord naturally falls off. During this time, the mother and baby bond and recuperate. Once the cord drops off, the newborn is introduced to close female relatives. A significant ritual called *'Sifudu'* involving smoke cleansing, is performed. Another important ritual, *'Inkaba'* is performed, which involves burying the baby's umbilical cord and afterbirth on ancestral grounds, symbolically connecting the child to their clan, ancestors and elders. Lastly, the *'Imbeleko'* ceremony welcomes the child into the broader community. This involves slaughtering a goat and inviting the clan to a feast, with the goat's skin becoming a sacred item for the new baby. In Xhosa culture, cattle and goats are sacred, representing the unity between the human material realm and the spiritual domain of universal gods and ancestors.

IN JAPAN, many women opt not to use pain medication during childbirth, influenced by Buddhist beliefs on suffering and that any pain endured during childbirth by the mother signifies her readiness for motherhood.

---

* *The Moiety System is a form of social organisation whereby society is divided into two complementary parts called 'moieties'. In many Indigenous cultures, there exists a belief in duality and that each half must come together to form a whole. This helps us to fully understand ourselves, the universe and out place within it.*

On the seventh night, a celebratory dinner marks the *'Oshichiya'* naming ceremony, where the father typically writes the baby's name and birthdate in calligraphy on white paper. For the first 21 days, the baby and mother stay at the maternal grandparents' house. At one-month-old, the baby participates in the *'Omiyamairi'* ceremony and visits a Shinto shrine, wearing a formal dress, where prayers for health and happiness are offered.

IN ANCIENT CHINESE TRADITION, the Zuo Yuezi Ritual, also known as *'Sitting the Month'* is observed by mothers following childbirth. Lasting for a moon cycle, this period entails confinement and adherence to special dietary restrictions, aiming to promote healing and replenish the mother's energy. According to Traditional Chinese Medicine, the initial three days post-birth focus on elimination, followed by 30 to 100 days of rest to restore lost blood and *Qi* energy from pregnancy and childbirth. During this time, ample physical rest is recommended, alongside tailored dietary plans to suit individual constitutional needs. Acupuncture and Traditional Chinese Medicine are integral components of postnatal care, helping to prevent and alleviate various postpartum issues such as depression, uterine bleeding and lactation difficulties. A notable practice, *'Mother Warming'* involves a one-time treatment performed four to five days after birth. This involves burning Mugwort to heat the abdomen, replenishing lost *Qi* energy and blood and aiding in postpartum recovery.

INUIT MOTHERING RITUALS encompass a variety of traditions and practices centred around childbirth and postpartum care. Traditionally, childbirth involved the attendance of a midwife and helpers who prepared a temporary bed in the woman's living space of a bush camp, teepee or house. After birth, the newborn was dried, wrapped in rabbit fur and cleaned, while the placenta, considered sacred, was carefully handled and either buried in the forest or hung in a tree. Breastfeeding immediately after delivery was customary for both practical and emotional bonding. A traditional cradle board, known as a *'tikinagan'* was common for safety and strengthening purposes, often incorporating moss as a natural nappy/diaper. Importance was placed on preserving the umbilical cord stump, which was considered sacred, usually kept in a moose hide and attached to the baby's bag for the child to play with. Postpartum care focuses on the mother's well-being, including isolation and natural remedies to promote recovery and support the family's overall health.

IN SLOVENIAN CULTURE, pregnancy and childbirth are surrounded by a tapestry of sacred customs, folklore practices and beliefs that honour the profound journey of bringing new life into the world. Throughout pregnancy, women refrain from cutting their hair, maintaining an unbroken connection with their unborn child. As childbirth approaches, women must keep their hair loose, enhancing the flow of energy and intuition and warding off negative energies. Ritual washing before delivery purifies the body and spirit. Fathers play an integral role, cleansing themselves spiritually after birth and presenting the newborn to nature's elements, raising the child to the sun, to the fire, laying them on the Earth and immersing them in a little water to symbolise the child's connection to the Divine. The placenta is buried under a tree and is watered with the first bath water. Protection against negative energies is sought through various means, such as drawing protective symbols or decorating cribs with red ribbons. Additionally, communal support is evident, with midwives receiving braided bread as a token of gratitude and families exchanging bread as a wish for perpetual abundance. These enduring rituals reflect a profound reverence for life and the interconnectedness of human existence with the natural world.

AS WE NAVIGATE the complexities of modern childbirth and postpartum care, there is much to be gleaned from the wisdom of indigenous traditions. By centring on indigenous knowledge and perspectives, we honour the diversity of human experience and open ourselves to a more holistic understanding of the postpartum journey. In doing so, we honour the wisdom of the past and pave the way for a future that embraces cultural diversity, respects ancestral traditions and nurtures the well-being of mothers and babies.

Attuned Parenting: Nurturing Connection and Resilience

Unlike rigid authoritarian or permissive styles, attuned parenting centres on understanding and responding to a child's emotional and developmental needs with profound empathy, fostering a deep sense of belonging and connection to the natural world, nervous system regulation and respectful relationships.

To embark on the journey of attuned parenting, one must first establish a solid foundation rooted in body wisdom and self-awareness so that one can develop the ability to recognise how one's mental and emotional state of being can profoundly impact one's child. Through attunement, you unlock the gateway to nurturing emotional intelligence, confidence and resilience in your children, providing them with the foundations for healthy social, emotional, and cognitive growth.

Central to the concept of attuned parenting is the modern philosophy of attachment parenting, popularised by pediatrician William Sears and his wife Martha Sears. This approach emphasises the cultivation of strong emotional bonds between caregivers and children through the practice of closeness. However, the modern world's stresses can challenge implementing attachment parenting principles. Babies inherently mirror the energy and emotions of their mothers through mirror neurons; thus, attachment parenting may fall short of addressing the complexities of modern stressors, leaving mothers feeling overwhelmed and inadequate despite their efforts, making attunement crucial.

Attuned parenting offers a remedy to this dilemma by empowering mothers to take ownership of their emotional state, energy expression and how they engage with their children and the impact it may have. Whilst most days it can feel like you are mostly surviving, prioritising self-regulation creates optimal environments where both mother and child can thrive. This journey toward attunement often requires the support and assistance of a supportive village community, which tells us what we already know, that no mother should be navigating parenthood alone.

It's worth noting the irony of modern language- in framing 'attachment parenting' as a novel concept when, historically and anthropologically speaking, it reflects Indigenous caregiving practices that have prevailed for generations. In our quest to decolonise birth and postpartum experiences, indigenous parenting, rooted in attunement to the needs of the child and the rhythms of nature, epitomises the essence of conscious parenting.

Indigenous cultures worldwide have long practiced a holistic approach to childcare, where infants are carried close to their caregivers, sleep alongside them and are breastfed on demand. These practices, deeply ingrained in the fabric of Indigenous communities, prioritise the well-being of both mother and child, fostering a sense of connection, security and belonging from the earliest stages of life.

In embracing the concept of attuned parenting, we recognise the profound impact of our presence, energy and responsiveness on our children's well-being and behaviours. By cultivating attunement, we nurture deep connections, resilience and flourishing for ourselves and our children, honouring the wisdom of primal caregiving practices while adapting to the realities of the modern world.

Cultural Babywearing: Celebrating Traditions Across Continents

Across diverse cultures worldwide, babywearing has been a cherished tradition, which helps to soothe distressed or tired babies, creating freedom of movement for mothers during daily life whilst maintaining secure attachments and nurturing the bond between mother and child.

In Aboriginal communities, mothers crafted carriers from paperbark or soft wood such as the *coolamon*, carrying babies close to the hip for easy transport. Throughout Africa, mothers used a length of fabric for the *traditional sling carry*, tying cloth over one shoulder and under the opposite arm for front or back carries. In the Americas, Inuit mothers kept their infants warm by wearing them within their coats, while various indigenous tribes, including Ojibwe, Navajo, Apache, Shoshone, Ute, Iroquois, Hopi, and Lakota, used cradleboards for safe transport, with variations in style and use across cultures.

In Japan, mothers wrap their babies in obi sashes or use the Onbuhimo carrying strap, which features a rectangle of fabric with straps at the top corners and loops at the bottom corners. Basket-style carriers were prevalent across Asia, as were soft structured carriers used by the Hmong hill tribes, whilst Central and South Americas used rebozos, and India utilised a baby sling hammock over the shoulder.

Modern Day Ergonomic Babywearing: Embracing Comfort and Connection

Today, babywearing focuses on prioritising the physical well-being and comfort of the wearer and the comfort and healthy development of the child. Central to this approach is the '*M position*', ensuring optimal hip alignment for the baby, promoting healthy development and preventing hip dysplasia. Modern ergonomic structured carriers feature designs with easy-to-secure buckles, padded straps and lower back support, enhancing comfort for the wearer during extended periods of use. The design of these carriers makes it easy for on-the-go parenting and adventures and are usually used for infants over 4 weeks old, or when they have gained the strength and ability to hold their heads up independently.

These carriers provide crucial support for the baby's head and neck, facilitate easy breastfeeding and promote upright, balanced posture for both parent and child. By distributing the baby's weight evenly and maintaining proper spine alignment, ergonomic baby carriers promote postpartum recovery and empower caregivers to engage in daily activities while nurturing their infants. Moreover, ergonomic babywearing fosters a sense of community and support among caregivers, celebrating the timeless bond between parent and child in a modern context.

Safe Co-Sleeping

Co-sleeping has been a cultural norm in many traditional societies, including various indigenous cultures and communities, fostering closeness and connection through shared sleeping spaces, with families gathering together on communal bedding. The practice of Co-sleeping extends beyond mere practicality though, as it serves as a symbol of nurturing and protection, where infants feel secure and loved in the presence of their caregivers.

Balancing Tradition with Safety

While co-sleeping has historical and cultural significance, modern caregivers must prioritise safety to ensure optimal infant conditions. Safe co-sleeping practices involve creating a sleep environment that minimises the risk of accidents or suffocation. This includes using a firm mattress with fitted sheets and removing soft bedding, pillows or other potential hazards from the sleeping area. Additionally, caregivers should avoid consuming alcohol, drugs or medications that may impair their awareness while co-sleeping. Positioning infants on their backs to sleep and ensuring they have their own separate sleep surface, such as a bassinet or co-sleeper attached to the adult bed can further reduce the risk of accidental suffocation or overlay. Moreover, maintaining a moderate room temperature and avoiding overheating infants with excessive clothing or bedding are essential safety considerations. By combining cultural traditions with evidence-based safety guidelines, caregivers can create a nurturing and secure co-sleeping environment that honours tradition and modern safety standards.

I CO-SLEPT with all four of my children. During the newborn days, I had them in bed with me, using a cosleeper and once we had established a strong breastfeeding connection, I moved them to a bassinet next to my bed, where I could reach over and soothe them during the night, patting them back to sleep. Once they had outgrown that, they were transitioned into a cot in the corner of the room. This helped me to respond to their needs quickly as I did not let my babies cry for too long.

I think it is important for babies to be able to sense and smell that their mother is close; they have spent many months inside your body, enveloped by your warmth and the rhythmic beating of your heart. Personally, I find it strange that we have been sold this idea that tiny babies need their own separate room, monitored by cameras, when we can have them close to us, helping their nervous system settle and their neurons be wired for safety and connection.

17

WOMB HEALING

NURTURING BODY AND SPIRIT POSTPARTUM

> "Her womb, once the cradle of life,
> now becomes the wellspring of her wisdom."
> -Donna Raymond

The most important thing to do after giving birth is to rest, relax and renew your Spirit. Your job now is to restore and replenish your body, which has just undergone a mammoth transition. If you've experienced surgery, your recovery time will be slightly longer. Allow the first few weeks to be solely about sacred imprinting, bonding with your baby, and getting to know your new mama's body, particularly if breastfeeding. It is really important to keep warm and support your womb to heal and restore itself.

Across cultures and holistic health traditions, the womb is a woman's wellness focal point, particularly in the transformative postpartum period. Revered as a sacred space symbolising the essence of womanhood and the source of life, the womb undergoes profound physical changes during pregnancy and childbirth. Beyond its physiological role, the womb is deeply intertwined with a woman's emotional and spiritual well-being, embodying ancestral wisdom passed down through generations. This holistic understanding recognises the importance of nurturing the womb for physical recovery and emotional and spiritual vitality, fostering a sense of connection to one's inner self, motherhood and ancestral lineage.

Incorporating ancient healing practices from traditions such as Traditional Chinese Medicine and Ayurveda, postpartum care emphasises the holistic balance of the womb's energy. From herbal remedies to abdominal massage and mindful practices like yoga and meditation, these approaches aim to restore harmony and vitality to the womb, supporting the woman's overall well-being. By honouring the womb as the centre of wellness, postpartum women embrace a profound journey of healing and renewal, guided by a deep reverence for the sacredness of their bodies and the wisdom of their ancestors.

Keep Warm

Remember to keep your womb warm, this will help foster healing. The cervix takes about 1 week to return to its natural size. The uterus typically takes about six weeks to return to its pre-pregnancy size postpartum. During this period, the uterus undergoes a process called involution, where it gradually shrinks back to its normal size and position. This process can vary slightly from woman to woman, but generally, most size reduction occurs within the first two weeks postpartum, with complete involution occurring by six weeks. If you have experienced abdominal surgery, your recovery time will be slightly longer. Remember, domestic duties can wait and it is totally okay for you to delegate tasks. If you are a strong, independent woman, it may be hard to ask for help, but there will be people around you willing and ready to serve you in this way.

Warmth is crucial for improving blood circulation, relaxing muscles, supporting the immune system and providing emotional comfort. It also helps prevent the invasion of cold, which can lead to issues like joint pain and digestive problems. Practical ways to keep warm include wearing layers of warm clothing and socks around the house, belly binding, womb steaming, consuming warm foods and drinks, taking warm baths, using heating pads and maintaining a warm living environment. Warmth relates to Ayurveda and Traditional Chinese Medicine principles, which are believed to promote the flow of vital energy and balance the body's energies.

The Art of Belly Binding

Belly binding, an age-old practice observed across diverse cultures, offers more than just physical recovery, it embodies a profound spiritual and emotional journey for women in the postpartum period. Known by various names like *sarashi, faja,* or *bengkung,* this tradition involves delicately wrapping the abdomen with cloth strips, imparting an array of health benefits that extend far beyond mere physical healing. From providing crucial support to core muscles and alleviating swelling to fostering better posture and relieving discomfort, belly binding is a testament to the holistic approach to postpartum care.

Embedded within belly binding is a rich tapestry of spiritual beliefs and cultural significance, serving as a vessel for honouring the divine feminine and embracing the sacredness of the postpartum experience. Through time-honoured rituals and ceremonies, women connect with their inner strength and wisdom, forging a deeper bond with their bodies and the miraculous journey of motherhood. This spiritual dimension nurtures emotional well-being and creates a sacred space for healing and reflection, allowing women to navigate the transition to motherhood with grace and empowerment.

For centuries, mothers across Asia, Europe, and Latin America have turned to belly binding as a trusted ally in their postpartum journey, recognising its efficacy in aiding weight loss, toning muscles and restoring abdominal integrity after childbirth.

As the abdomen contracts and the cloth tightens, it symbolises physical transformation and the resilience and beauty of the female body. Embracing belly binding transcends mere physical recovery, it is a powerful celebration of motherhood, weaving together tradition, spirituality and profound healing on the sacred path of nurturing new life.

Women should be wrapped as soon they can after birth, ideally on day five postpartum. The belly bind should be worn for 10-12 hours a day for at least 40 days or longer. After a cesarean birth, women should wait at least 6 weeks until the incision is mostly healed before they are wrapped.

As with all things, listen to your body and what feels right for you. I wrapped my belly after all three of my home births, though I did not do it with the traditional knotted style. For me, I purchased a decent length of material in a cotton lycra blend, as I needed to be able to adjust it due to the nature of my back pain from past accidents. It still worked the same and what was interesting is that my body couldn't tolerate it being too tight to give the flat effect you see in the traditional belly binds. I would experience a very sharp stabbing pain in my womb, would get the sweats and feel dizzy and lightheaded. I had minor *diastasis recti* *after giving birth the third time. I wore my wrap daily until bedtime for the first 2.5 weeks and every other day for 1 month.

POP- Breaking the Silence of Pelvic Organ Prolapse

Pelvic Organ Prolapse (*POP*) is a condition that many new mothers experience, yet it often remains shrouded in silence and misunderstanding. The physical and emotional demands of childbirth can lead to changes in the body that are unexpected and *POP* is one of those changes that occur when the muscles and tissues supporting the pelvic organs; such as the bladder, uterus or rectum, become weakened or stretched. This can lead to one or more of these organs slipping out of their normal positions and pressing into, or even out of, the vaginal canal. There are different forms of prolapse, including *cystocele*, where the bladder drops into the front wall of the vagina; *rectocele*, when the rectum bulges into the back wall of the vagina; and *uterine prolapse*, when the uterus descends into or through the vagina. Prolapse can range from mild to severe, with some women experiencing no symptoms and others finding it impacts their daily lives.

Childbirth is one of the most common causes of prolapse. The intense pressure and strain placed on the pelvic floor muscles during pregnancy and birth can lead to weakening or injury. Vaginal birth, espe-

---

* *Diastasis Recti is a condition where the large abdominal muscles separate.*

cially with a large baby, prolonged labour, or instrumental delivery (using forceps or vacuum), is a significant risk factor. Multiple births can further weaken the pelvic floor with each pregnancy and chronic straining from conditions such as constipation, chronic cough, or heavy lifting can exacerbate the problem.

Recognising the signs of *POP* is crucial for early intervention and treatment. Symptoms to be aware of include a feeling of heaviness or pressure in the pelvis, often described as a sensation of *'something falling out'*; discomfort or pain during intercourse, urinary issues like difficulty emptying the bladder, frequent urination, or incontinence; bowel problems such as constipation or a feeling of incomplete emptying and in some cases, a visible or palpable bulge in the vaginal area. If you experience any of these symptoms, it's important to consult with a healthcare provider for a proper diagnosis.

Overcoming the shame associated with *POP* is vital part to the healing process. The stigma surrounding prolapse can leave many women feeling embarrassed or isolated, but it's essential to recognise that *POP* is a common condition. Studies suggest that between 30% to 50% of women who have given birth will experience some degree of pelvic organ prolapse[1] There is no shame in experiencing prolapse, and seeking help is a powerful step towards healing. By speaking openly about *POP*, we can break down the barriers of silence and support one another in the postnatal journey. Understanding that prolapse is a natural consequence of the immense physical effort involved in bringing new life into the world can help diminish feelings of guilt or inadequacy.

While *POP* can be challenging, there are effective treatments and strategies to manage and improve symptoms. Strengthening the pelvic floor muscles through regular exercises can help alleviate mild prolapse and prevent further progression. Physical therapy, guided by a pelvic floor specialist can provide tailored exercises and manual therapy to support recovery. Pessaries, which are devices inserted into the vagina to support the pelvic organs, can offer relief from symptoms, and lifestyle modifications, such as managing weight, avoiding heavy lifting and treating chronic cough or constipation, can reduce strain on the pelvic floor. In more severe cases, surgery may be recommended to repair the prolapse and restore normal function.

Vaginal Hydrotherapy

In the delicate postpartum period, new mothers often seek holistic approaches to healing that nurture both their physical and spiritual well-being. *Vaginal hydrotherapy*, also known as womb or pelvic steaming, emerges as a revered practice across cultures, offering comprehensive healing for women in the postpartum phase. This ancient tradition involves sitting over a steaming pot of water infused with medicinal herbs, gently permeating the vaginal and pelvic region. Beyond its physical benefits, postpartum vaginal hydrotherapy holds profound spiritual significance, offering new mothers a sacred space for emotional release and renewal as they navigate the transition to motherhood.

Postpartum vaginal hydrotherapy offers a myriad of physical benefits, making it a powerful tool for postpartum recovery. Firstly, the herbal steam promotes circulation to the pelvic area, aiding in healing and reducing inflammation and swelling associated with childbirth. The steam's warmth can relieve postpartum discomforts such as cramps and pelvic pain. Moreover, vaginal hydrotherapy supports the toning and tightening of the pelvic floor muscles, enhancing bladder control and promoting overall pelvic health. By detoxifying the pelvic region, this practice can also assist in hormonal balance and contribute to reproductive wellness.

Beyond its physical effects, postpartum vaginal hydrotherapy holds deep spiritual significance, providing new mothers with a sacred space for emotional healing and connection. This ancient ritual becomes a transformative act of self-care and self-love, allowing women to release any emotional traumas or blockages accumulated during childbirth. Through the nurturing warmth of the herbal steam, women can tap into their innate wisdom, intuition and feminine power, fostering a deeper connection to themselves and their role as mothers.

Before you begin your pelvic steaming journey, I highly encourage you to seek out a practitioner for a personal consultation so that they can create a steam protocol that is specific to your body's needs, as the amount of time and herbs used can vary. I say this because after my fourth born, I treated myself to a postpartum consultation and the wisdom I received and the protocol made for me completely changed my postpartum experience and recovery time.

How to prepare your Pelvic Steam.

1. **Prepare the Steam:** Bring a pot of water to a gentle boil and add a blend of medicinal herbs such as rosemary, lavender, calendula and chamomile. Allow the herbs to steep for several minutes, infusing the water with their healing properties.
2. **Set the Scene:** Create a calm and comfortable space for your vaginal hydrotherapy session. Choose a quiet room where you can relax and unwind without distractions, set up an area for your baby to be near you if needed.
3. **Position Yourself:** Sit comfortably over the pot of steaming herbal water, ensuring that you are a safe distance away to avoid burns. Use a stool or chair with a hole in the seat for support. Please make sure this is made of natural materials and is unvarnished.
4. **Cover Yourself:** Drape a blanket or large towel around your waist and over your lower body to create a tent-like enclosure, trapping the steam and directing it towards the vaginal and pelvic area.
5. **Engage in Mindfulness:** Close your eyes and focus on your breath as you allow the herbal steam to envelop you. Visualise the healing warmth penetrating your body, releasing tension and promoting relaxation. Use this sacred time to reflect on your journey as a mother and what your needs are.
6. **Stay Hydrated:** Drink plenty of water before and after your vaginal hydrotherapy session to stay hydrated and support the detoxification process.
7. **Listen to Your Body:** Pay attention to any sensations or discomfort during the session, adjusting the temperature or

duration of the steam as needed to ensure your comfort and safety.
8. **Rest and Reflect:** After your vaginal hydrotherapy session, take time to rest and reflect on your experience. Journaling or meditation can be beneficial for processing any emotions that arise during the healing process

BY EMBRACING THIS ANCIENT TRADITION, women tap into their innate vitality, wisdom and feminine power, reclaiming their bodies and honouring the transformative journey of motherhood. Through the ritual of vaginal hydrotherapy, women emerge strengthened, empowered and renewed, embodying the sacred essence of the divine feminine as they navigate the beautiful path of motherhood.

Closing of the Bones

The *Closing of the Bones* ritual is a deeply restorative, sacred postpartum practice with roots in various traditional cultures, particularly in Central and South America. This ancient ritual honours the new mother and helps her transition from the intense process of childbirth to a phase of healing and restoration. The ritual involves wrapping the mother's body with cloth or scarves, especially the abdomen, hips, and chest. This gentle yet firm wrapping helps to physically support and realign the mother's body, which has expanded and shifted to accommodate childbirth. The wrapping aids in bringing the bones and organs back to their pre-pregnancy positions, providing physical support and stability, alleviating discomfort and promoting faster recovery of the body's musculoskeletal system.

Closing of the Bones is also a time for emotional and psychological healing. The ritual creates a sacred space where the new mother can process her birth experience, release any trauma and embrace her new identity. The nurturing touch and presence of the practitioner provide a sense of being held and cared for, which is crucial for emotional well-being. This practice can help mitigate feelings of vulnerability and overwhelm, fostering a sense of closure and completeness.

The ritual helps to seal the birth field, grounding and centring the new mother. This can restore a sense of wholeness and balance, aligning the body, mind and spirit. The ritual often includes elements such as massage, herbal treatments, and the use of warming oils, all of which contribute to the energetic rebalancing and overall sense of well-being. Often performed by a skilled practitioner, such as a midwife or doula, the ritual can involve family members as a reminder that the new mother is not alone and has a support system. This communal aspect is empowering and reinforces the importance of community in the postpartum period. Through this ancient ritual, mothers can find closure, strength and a renewed sense of self as they embark on their journey of motherhood.

Acknowledgement and Sealing Ceremony

Birth is such an incredibly intimate journey for all women. It is something special and Sacred and as unique as each baby and mother born to this process.

As birth opens you, stretching you wide in full surrender to the Great Mystery, there must be space held for this new Mother identity to come back fully into your body, for your Spirit to settle and feel nourished. To return home. A place to realise that birth as an initiation has come to completion and you are now on the other side of birth's doorstep, as a mother, forever changed.

The concept of *'sealing'* relates to the integration process of any initiation. Once you've completed the inner work, gained insight and are ready to implement necessary changes or embody a new state of being.

Creating a Sacred Ceremonial space is paramount to your physical, mental, emotional and spiritual health and wellbeing postpartum. It creates the space for you to be in a moment that sits outside of time, a time to connect with, reflect upon and gather all the pieces of yourself and bring them into the present moment, claiming your new role as Mother, welcoming and accepting all the changes that have taken place and that are coming. It is absolutely necessary to prioritise this space for yourself, in a way that uplifts and inspires you into your power. It does not need to be an elaborate ritual, and in all honesty, sometimes the most profound moments can come from simplicity. What is required though is quiet space where you feel calm, relaxed and fully supported to collect yourself, all parts, so that you come to acceptance and completion of your birthing journey. It is important to be with the raw, real emotions as they move through your body. Be with the grief and the joy, the clarity and the confusion. Both can exist at the same time and can be felt with deep honesty as you come to terms with the enormity of the initiation you've just journeyed through. You need to create a safe space for you to integrate and land back in your body.

Sealing Ceremonial Bath

A sealing ceremonial bath will help you to create a powerful ritual to acknowledge the journey of birthing, soaking in the wisdom you have garnerd through introspection.

Using candles, herbs, flowers and ritual oils you create a sacred space to cleanse and renew your spirit. You can also write powerful words of affirmation on your skin, speak your incantations and prayers into the water and soften into the beauty you have created for yourself. Alternatively, you can seek spaces in Nature whether salt or freshwater to immerse your whole body to cleanse and renew. In this way, you can wash away what no longer serves and emerge lifted and gifted with a new awareness from your healing.

If you don't have a bath, it will serve you well to ask a friend, hire a place or have a simple foot bath if that is all you have access to. It needs to be private, safe and warm.

Water is healing, it is deeply symbolic of the emotional realms and the subconscious. As an element, water connects us to the power and force of change and natural lore. It helps to nourish and sustain us. We are made up of over 80% water, so bathing in a body of warm water can help us connect with our Soul's truth and the essence of who we are, beyond the stories and challenges that life presents us with.

With any ceremony, intention and presence is key, so make sure that as you are preparing your Sacred space, lighting candles, incense, diffusing essential oils etc, you do so with awareness of what this is all for. This is for you, dear woman, beautiful Mother.

As you draw your bath, call in any spiritual deities and devas that you connect with. Call in the Great Mother and allow her primal energy to imbue your space with love and understanding. You might like to add milk and honey to your bath, if you are using honey, I suggest you use Manuka for its medicinal and healing properties- this will help if you have had a perineum tear. If you are wanting to work with essential oils make sure you use a dispersing agent like pure castile soap or a carrier oil, so the oils do not sit on the surface of the water and irritate your skin. You can also add the oils into a cup of whole milk and then add to your bath. It is important not to add oils to hot water as they will evaporate and so with the therapeutic qualities and benefits the oils bring.

Add herbs and flower petals if you feel called to, bring in anything from your birthing space into the sealing ceremony, so that you can connect with the birthing field and begin to close down these portals.

Preparing any type of ceremonial drink, like a comforting tea will help you relax into the space, and drop deeper into the moment of reflection and integration.

Working with your essential oils when you are in the natural hormonal high of postpartum can be beneficial to aromatically anchor those emotions and feelings, so that when a rough day comes to pass, and there will be many, you can reach for you oils to support and serve as a reminder of how incredibly powerful you are.

Consider using relaxing floral botanicals like lavender, jasmine, rose, geranium, clary sage, ylang ylang, neroli, sandalwood ginger, vetiver and frankincense.

Placenta: The Tree of Life

The placenta is a unique vascular organ that receives blood supplies from both the maternal and the fetal systems and thus has two separate circulatory systems for blood: the maternal-placental (*uteroplacental*) blood circulation, and the fetal-placental (*fetoplacental*) blood circulation. Both contribute cells to form the organ, a disk that usually measures around 8 inches in diameter and weighs about a pound by the time a baby is born. The fetal side is smooth and glistening, with a pronounced network of branching blood vessels, sometimes nicknamed the tree of life. The placenta is a key site of spiritual meaning for some birthing women, embodying the link between woman, child and the transformation of pregnancy and birth

Birthing blood is Sacred and there is no escaping the messiness that birth brings with it. You may notice tinges of blood in your 'show' or you may have a bloody show on transition. Blood is a natural part of birth and it is important to claim this blood for ritual purposes because it is incredibly powerful.

The best way to collect your blood is to be prepared to birth the placenta into a bowl. For my 2 waterbirths once I had brought my baby up to my heart to claim them, I waited a few minutes and then got out of the bath to birth the placenta. A big reason for this is because I was borderline anaemic and so had a high risk of haemorrhaging, so being outside of the bath would allow me to monitor the amount of blood loss. I had a large stainless steel bowl ready and simply knelt or squat over it whilst bringing baby to breast to stimulate oxytocin and contractions to birth the placenta. Within 15min a healthy placenta was released. It can take longer for some women, if this is the case do whatever you can to stay relaxed and continue stimulating the oxytocin.

When the womb clamps down and expels the placenta, there is a gush of blood that accompanies and it feels AMAZING!!!

> -*"In term infants, one-minute delay in cord clamping after birth leads to an additional 80 mL of blood from the placenta to the infant's circulation, which increases to about 100 mL by 3 minutes after birth."*[2]

Let the placenta sit for a while so that baby is getting all those potent stem cells and then drain any excess birthing blood and store it into a vessel of personal significance. I used a beautiful ceramic vase I had made in art school. Place this dark womab blood in the fridge if you want to use for any ritual ceremonies later. Otherwise mix with water and feed your favourite plants.

This is sacred blood, treat it as such.

Lotus Birth

The deep spiritual philosophy behind Lotus birthing is that it is not up to us to sever the connection between baby and mother, rather it is up to the newborn child to choose when they're ready to let go. It is the ultimate extension of gentle birth and Sovereignty foundations.

All three of my daughters were semi-lotus births. That meant that I birthed my baby and then placenta, leaving the umbilical cord intact, hoping to fall away in due time (complete lotus) only that was not the case for me.

I must digress though that living in the tropics meant it was a little challenging to navigate lotus birth and with each birth the chances of having an undisturbed bonding time postpartum diminished with the the needs of an inquisitive and active toddler. So for full clarity my lotus births were not totally complete.

Auraura Freedom's cord was hanging on by a thread on day 4 and was irritating her so much that we decided to cut the dried-out umbilical stalk so that it could sit in her cloth nappy more easily. It fell off completely in the bath the next day.

Maia Lily was much the same, only I was more experienced and prepared with a beautiful placenta bag that a close sister had made for me. On day 3 her name came through clearly and once her name was spoken in ceremony, I tuned in to see if it was ok and with the all clear from Spirit...decided to chew the dried out umbilical with my teeth. It was incredibly tough and hard to chew through, it felt completely primal and natural to do this, mind you I'm pretty sure it freaked her paternal grandmother out!

As Lucah Belle was born in the peak of a hot Australian summer, I had full intentions to lotus, though she was born in a heat wave so there were plenty of flies buzzing around (my house is totally open). I bled the placenta and then around 3-4hrs later, when her cord was rubbery and clear we tied it with hemp twine and cut it at around 10cm from the connection to her abdomen. Zenith's was much the same.

Natural Lotus birthing is not for everyone, but for those that are interested, it is much easier to do in a homebirth setting. With respects to birthing inside an establishment like public/private hospital or birthing centre, you will need to discuss this with staff before hand, as each facility will have different protocols for handling what they call *'bio-waste'* which is what your placenta will be classed as. When I gave birth to Auraura, I had the first lotus birth at the Mareeba Birthing Centre in North Queensland. My midwife fetched me a clean 4L icecream container to place the placenta into. I had spoken to her about my desire to have a lotus birth but was actually unprepared, so was grateful even though it was incredibly awkward. I'm so glad I did it. When we went to discharge from the hospital 5 days later, I had to sign a release/waiver form to keep the placenta and took it home frozen.

Placenta Preparation and Curing

You will need to bleed placenta for 24hrs. To do this you can place the placenta into a colander or veggie steamer with pot underneath to catch excess fluids. Cover with a sprinkle of salt to encourage the excess fluid to drain and any aromatic herbs or flowers of your choice and then place lid on or a cloth over the top.

You will need to keep baby rather still for the first 24hrs as you bleed the placenta and as awkward as it seems, find your groove breastfeeding. Sometimes the cord can feel cold and sticky so keep that in mind. You might like to keep some extra muslin wraps close by.

After you've collected the first initial bleed, notice how much the placenta has shrunk in size. Place this sacred blood into a different container and label it. I put mine in an old glass coffee jar and placed in the fridge to use in placenta blessing ceremonies. Pat down the plancenta of any excess fluid, rinse it if it starts to smell and then redress with a sprinkle of salt and aromatic herbs. The salt and herbs are what help to dehydrate and cure the placenta.

Aim for minimal disturbance. Keep checking the placenta and cord to make sure it is kept clean. If done correctly, there should be no smell. There should be no foul smelling odour or rotting flesh. The cord will begin to dry out completely and detach itself around day 3-5 and depending on child and environmental conditions, could last up to 10days.

Consuming Placenta

Preparing the placenta for consumption by mothers is considered traditional among Vietnamese and Chinese people. The Chinese believe a nursing mother should boil the placenta, make a broth and then drink it to improve her milk

There are a few different ways you can consume your placenta if you feel called to. Most animals consume the afterbirth, both as a way to limit the scent of birth that would bring in potential predators and to restore the body with vital nutrients the mother lost during pregnancy and birth.

Today, most women who subscribe to this belief will encapsulate their placenta to consume in the days after birth, when their immune system or their hormones and emotions need support. If this is something you wish to consider, there are plenty of resources available online to help you prepare. I did not do this personally so can not share what I feel is the best recipe, however I do believe that you should consider outsourcing and get someone to do it for you, so you can stay in the sacred bubble of postpartum.

Eating Raw Placenta

This was the option that I took after Maia Lily was born. Interestingly enough, because she was still attached to her placenta after I bled it for 24 hours, I was called to rip a 20-cent-sized piece off from the Mother's side. The moment when I tore the flesh, Maia had a reflex response. It's incredible how we can often think that the lifeless cord and placenta are not energetically attached to the baby.

With that small piece, I ripped it up into 6 smaller ones and froze. You could blend them up in a smoothie if you wanted to, I simply swallowed it whole and because it was frozen and there was no taste.

I can not tell you exactly why I was called to do it in this way, It came through my womb and I simply listened and honoured it, like I do with all wisdom that comes through me in this way. I can put my rational spin on it in that when I became a mother for the first time I had a STRONG AND CLEAR message come through me that all placentas are meant to be returned to the Earth. That is a big reason why I took a small piece, enough to fulfil my needs and not take from creating a sense of belonging for my new daughter.

Returning the Placenta to the Great Mother

In my *dreaming*, I was given a strong message from the Great Mother, calling for placentas to be returned to the land. I was 22 when I transitioned from *Maiden to Mother* and didn't understand the significance of this message. I just did what I was told.

Returning the placenta to the Earth helps to anchor a deep spiritual connection to the land and Mother. It fosters a fundamental sense of belonging and allows the Spirit of the child to rest in knowing that they are secure in their sense of place. Ideally, the placenta is ceremoniously buried where the baby is born, their homeland.

Following the wisdom and guidance from Spirit, I facilitated a sacred blessing ceremony for my children, which called in the surrounding community to provide them with blessings for their journey through life. I felt that this was important because it takes a village to raise a child and it is beautiful when the child gets to experience the love and support from those around them, to know that they are held and that they matter, even if they are an infant, the imprint runs deep.

I buried all of my placentas under a tree. Auraua had an Orange tree and Maia had a Rolinia, but it died, so I planted a lemon tree in the same spot. Lucah had a Lychee tree and Zenith had an Evodia, which is the food plant for the Ulysses butterfly.

If you're worried about the longevity of your homelands, you can always bury your placenta with a potted plant and that way you can take it with you wherever you roam and gift it to your child during a coming of age ceremony, or perhaps once they are mature and settling in their own place. Alternatively, you can bury the placenta in a sacred place close to your heart where you have a special connection to the land, ancestral ties or family story.

18

THE ART OF BREASTFEEDING
A JOURNEY OF NOURISHMENT, WISDOM AND TRANSITION

"Breastfeeding reminds us of the universal truth of abundance; the more we give out, the more we are filled up, and that divine nourishment - the source from which we all draw is, like a mother's breast, ever full and ever flowing."
-Sara Buckley

Breasts are such incredible and wondrous things. Unfortunately, our society has over-sexualised this important body part and has shamed the natural functions that are designed to nurture and provide life-giving nutrients to your young.

As you journey through pregnancy, you will notice that your breasts begin to change. They may start to feel more sensitive and even lumpy. This is all normal as your breasts begin to develop the milk ducts that will produce and store the milk that feeds your baby. Your areolas will darken in colour and change shape and size. My areolas went from peachy to almost purplish-brown by about 6 months gestation with my first child.

As you begin to ripen, you may start noticing the sticky yellow/orangish liquid that is secreted from your nipples. This incredibly potent and nutrient-dense liquid gold is called colostrum and will become your baby's first feed. It is loaded with goodness that prepares the baby's immune system and prepares them for life outside the womb. Your breasts function on the primal wisdom of supply and demand. They can also help to regulate your baby's body temperature and provide nurturing when your baby is overstimulated or needs the safety and comfort of mama.

Never forget that you are your baby's whole world. They sense your smells and emotions. I realised early on that breastfeeding was an incredibly spiritual and sacred journey of bonding between my daughter and I and did everything as naturally as possible, including curing a nasty bout of mastitis. Yes, it was challenging sometimes, but it was ultimately worth it.

Breastfeeding Facts

- Breast size doesn't necessarily correlate with milk production. Smaller breasts can produce just as much milk as larger ones.
- Breast milk is uniquely tailored to the specific nutritional needs of the baby at different stages of development and can happen whilst tandem nursing.
- Nursing will burn a significant number of calories. Producing breastmilk consumes 25% of the body's energy, the brain only uses 20%!
- There are 3 stages of milk production in the first few weeks postpartum: colostrum, transitional milk and mature milk.
- Breast milk contains antibodies and stem cells that help protect infants from infections and illnesses, boosting their immune systems.
- Mothers who breastfeed have a reduced long-term risk of cardiovascular disease, diabetes and breast and ovarian cancer. The longer the duration of breastfeeding the greater the reduction in risk of disease. [1]
- According to the American Academy of Pediatrics, breastfeeding enhances children's neurodevelopmental outcomes and improves their long-term physical and dental health. It also significantly reduces the risk of various medical

conditions, including SIDS, asthma, diabetes and leukemia. Additionally, breastfeeding benefits maternal health by lowering the risk of certain cancers, type 2 diabetes, hypertension and postpartum depression.
- Nursing triggers the release of oxytocin, often called the 'love hormone' that promotes bonding between mother and baby. Oxytocin helps with uterine contractions post-birth, can reduce bleeding and help the uterus return to its pre-pregnancy size more quickly. It also triggers the release of endorphins in both mother and baby, providing natural pain relief and is linked to lower rates of postpartum depression.
- Prolactin, the breastfeeding hormone helps mothers feel more relaxed and emotionally stable, enhancing their patience and responsiveness to their baby's needs.
- Unlike formula feeding, breastfeeding doesn't require bottles or formula, making it a more efficient and environmentally sustainable choice.
- Expressed breastmilk can be safely stored at room temperature for up to 4 hours and then refrigerated or frozen to preserve nutritional quality.
- Some women experience colostrum leakage, a precursor to breast milk, during pregnancy. This can happen as early as the second trimester.
- 75% of women produce more milk in their right breast.
- Breasts can detect even a one-degree fluctuation in a baby's body temperature. The temperature of breast milk adjusts according to the baby's needs, offering warmth or hydration as needed; that's why skin-to-skin contact is crucial in the early days.
- Breastfeeding mothers and babies may synchronise their biological clocks, with mothers often experiencing a 'let down' of milk before their baby cries for a feed.
- Breastfeeding saves a family approximately $1200-$2000 annually compared to the cost of formula.

Breastfeeding Wisdom

When babies are born, their stomachs are the size of a pea or a small stonefruit. We produce colostrum first because it is a small amount of nutrient-dense liquid that establishes a normal gut microbiome; that's why it's called *'Liquid Gold'*. Our bodies are perfectly equipped to nurture our children, although there are some rare occasions where some women are physiologically unable to breastfeed due to medical reasons and other factors.

In my years of mothering and listening to women's stories, I realised there was a startling number of women who were not given adequate education about this incredibly sacred experience. It made me sad to know that so many women stopped breastfeeding between 2-6 weeks because it was too hard, or they thought their body wasn't producing enough milk. So, I want to share everything I've learned from my almost 8 years of breastfeeding.

Supply and Demand

Once your baby is born, follow the prompts and signals that they are hungry. Do not follow a timer. Follow your baby's natural rhythm for hunger. As your milk comes in, it can be quite painful and uncomfortable. Remedies to help soothe sore and engorged breasts include the age-old use of whole cabbage leaves to cup the breasts, warm compress and gentle massage (only enough to elevate the engorgement).

If you find that your breasts are painfully engorged, do not play with them, as it can stimulate your supply. I made this mistake with my first baby, as I was fully engorged and in pain. I was encouraged to massage and express some milk out in a warm shower because my breasts were so engorged you could hardly see the point of the nipple. It was too hard to feed. So away I went, happily expressing because it felt so good to relieve the pressure but I paid for it the next day because my breasts were EVEN BIGGER!!! The moral of the story, remember the law of supply and demand. If you feel you are not producing enough milk, this can work in your favour to help boost supply.

. . .

Your milk will transition through a series of changes and you may notice that at these times, your baby is super fussy, perhaps constantly on and off the breast, whingey or maybe even frustrated. When this happens, you need to keep feeding as much as possible, whenever you can as it will help increase your supply.

You will know that you are producing enough milk by the output, that is, how many wet/soiled nappies your baby has and it is the best indicator of your supply. For newborns, you want around 10 wet nappies a day. Don't be too concerned if they don't move their bowels for a few days, even up to a week, as it means they use every last bit of nutrition to service a growth spurt. If they are uncomfortable, you can massage their belly to encourage a bowel movement, especially if they might be a little backed up from a change of milk and perhaps dehydrated.

Emptying the breast is another key factor in maintaining your milk supply. Make sure your baby empties one breast before switching to the other side. Emptying the breast signals your body to produce more milk. Additionally, skin-to-skin contact with your baby can help stimulate milk production and promote bonding. Spend time cuddling with your baby without clothing barriers, especially during feedings.

Using a breast pump after nursing can further stimulate milk production. Pumping for a few minutes after each nursing session can help increase milk supply over time.

Staying hydrated is crucial, so drink plenty of fluids throughout the day. Aim for at least 8-10 glasses of water or other hydrating beverages daily.

One of the highlights of my breastfeeding journey was being able to support other mothers in feeding their children by becoming a milk donor. Initially, I contacted the two local hospitals, thinking I could donate my excess milk to mothers who had their supply disrupted, but unfortunately, they did not accept donations. So I used some of this milk to mix with food when introducing solids and donating the other directly to mothers who needed it. In 2007, this wasn't that common in my local area, though times have changed since then, and these days, there are more community efforts of human milk banks where mothers can access this liquid gold.

I have supported several mothers and babies with my excess milk. I never charged for my milk, though some women do to earn extra income. I only donated what I could without putting too much pressure on myself to become a milk machine. Sometimes that was 300ml, other times it was 30ml, and all were graciously received with gratitude.

Boosting and Maintaining Milk Supply

The most crucial aspects of increasing milk production are hydration, frequent nursing, restorative sleep and reducing stress. The more often you nurse your baby, the more signals your body receives to produce milk, basic supply and demand

Ensure that your baby is latched correctly and nursing effectively. A proper latch helps stimulate milk production and ensures your baby gets enough milk. If you're unsure about the latch or have any concerns with breastfeeding in general, consult with a *Thompson Method Breastfeeding Educator* or an *International Board Certified Lactation Consultant* as early as possible. They will support you to develop trust in your ability to nurse and work with your baby to establish a long-term breastfeeding relationship. If you notice a weak latch, milk starts to dribble from the corners of the mouth as your baby feeds, they pull on and off the nipple, or you hear a clicking sound, seek professional help to check for oral ties as these can hinder the success of long-term breastfeeding.

Maintaining a balanced and nutritious diet is essential for milk production. Include plenty of fruits, vegetables, whole grains, lean proteins and healthy fats in your meals. Some foods, like oatmeal and certain herbs known as *galactagogues*, are believed to help boost milk supply.

Prioritise rest and relaxation as much as possible as cortisol, the stress hormone, can negatively impact milk supply. Take breaks when needed, practice deep breathing or meditation and enlist the help of supportive friends and family members. If you're struggling to increase your milk supply, seek help from a lactation consultant, breastfeeding support group, or healthcare provider.

Natural Remedies

1. **Water**: Staying hydrated is essential for milk production. Make sure to drink plenty of good quality water throughout the day to support lactation. Keep a water bottle in your bag and at your feeding station and drink at least a glass of water each time you nurse.
2. **Oatmeal:** Besides being a key ingredient in lactation cookies, oatmeal is known to help increase milk production. Have it for breakfast or as an easy go-to snack.
3. **Fenugreek**: Commonly used to boost milk supply. It can be consumed in supplement form or added to foods as a spice.
4. **Fennel:** This is believed to stimulate milk production. You can incorporate fennel seeds into your diet by adding them to dishes or brewing them into a tea.
5. **Barley:** Is rich in beta-glucan, which is thought to enhance lactation. Add to soups, stews or salads for a nutritious boost.
6. **Blessed Thistle:** An herb traditionally used to increase milk production in nursing mothers. It is often combined with fenugreek in lactation supplements.
7. **Alfalfa:** Is rich in vitamins and minerals and is believed to support lactation. It can be consumed as a tea or by adding sprouts to salads and sandwiches.
8. **Goat's Rue:** This has been used for centuries to stimulate milk production. It can be taken as a supplement or brewed into tea.
9. **Milk Thistle:** Commonly used to support liver health, it may also positively affect milk production. It can be taken as a supplement or brewed into tea.
10. **Marshmallow Root:** Thought to have lactogenic properties and may help increase milk supply. It can be brewed into tea or taken as a supplement.
11. **Motherwort:** In addition to its potential role in increasing milk supply, motherwort is also used to support cardiovascular health, reduce anxiety and stress and regulate menstrual cycles.

Lactation Cookies

Brewers Yeast is often the main ingredient in lactation recipes due to its reputation for supporting milk production. Rich in B vitamins and minerals like chromium and selenium, it's believed to help boost energy levels and milk supply. You can incorporate Brewers Yeast into lactation cookies and smoothies or sprinkle it over oatmeal for an added nutritional boost. However, if you have a sensitivity to yeast or experience any adverse reactions, it's advisable to consult with a healthcare professional before consuming it as a lactation aid.

Ingredients:

- 1 cup unsalted butter, softened
- 1 cup granulated sugar
- 1 cup brown sugar, packed
- 4 tablespoons brewer's yeast
- 2 tablespoons ground flaxseed meal
- 2 large eggs
- 1 teaspoon vanilla extract
- 2 cups all-purpose flour
- 1 teaspoon baking soda
- 1 teaspoon salt
- 3 cups old-fashioned oats
- 1 cup chocolate chips or raisins (optional)

Instructions:

1. Preheat your oven to 180 degrees Celsius. Line a baking tray with baking paper.
2. In a large mixing bowl, cream the butter, granulated sugar and brown sugar until smooth.
3. Add brewer's yeast, ground flaxseed meal, eggs and vanilla extract into the mixture. Beat until well combined.
4. In a separate bowl, whisk together the flour, baking soda and salt.

5. Gradually add the dry ingredients to the wet ingredients, mixing until just combined.
6. Fold in the oats and chocolate chips or raisins.
7. Using a spoon or cookie scoop, drop tablespoon-sized portions of dough onto the prepared baking sheet, spacing them about 2 inches apart.
8. Bake in the preheated oven for 10-12 minutes, or until the cookies are golden brown around the edges.
9. Allow the cookies to cool on the baking sheet for a few minutes before transferring them to a wire rack to cool completely. Enjoy.

My Breastfeeding Initiation

My initiation into breastfeeding my firstborn was quite rough. I went from barely filling an A cup to DD's overnight. All those years wishing I had big boobs answered, but the novelty soon wore off. On day 5 postpartum, my milk came in; I had cleavage up to my collar bones and was painfully engorged with itchy purple stretchmarks.

The sensations of my 'let down' were painful, and I would release up to 150ml of foremilk like a fountain. I was drowning my daughter as she tried to keep up with the explosive flow of milk. She would cough and splutter, and it took me a couple of days to realise it was better to express the letdown into a bowl or towel and then latch her to my breast when the flow wasn't as intense. This was quite hard to do when I had a screaming, hungry baby, desperate for 'susu'.*

I didn't go out much and it took around 6months for my breasts to calm down! I was bursting with milk. Everywhere. Drenching bras and bedsheets, the moist environment of the rainforest coupled with sticky, milk-soaked bras, shirts and sheets meant I had created the perfect little microclimate for thrush to thrive.

Feeding became painful, with stabbing pains through my nipples. My areola's paled in pigment and my daughter's tongue developed a thick coating of white. After battling to get nilstat drops into her mouth

---

* Susu is a term for the female breast or breastmilk.

and rubbing sticky daktarin gel on my nipples, washing my clothes constantly, I finally got it under control. She was a colicky baby who screamed for what felt like the first 8months of her life.

In the early days, I would just feed her when she cried; she was desperate for comfort, but this only added to the problem. Poor thing probably had severe indigestion and after hours of her screaming and walking the floor, I'd finally get her to settle and she'd be hungry again. This cycle repeated for months.

I'll never forget a quite poignant moment of sheer and utter defeat. It was around 3 am, it was cold and we had a rough week with hardly any sleep or reprieve. I was so highly strung. She was screaming. I had changed, fed her as usual and walked around with her in my arms, with my eyes closed. I had mapped the floor and counted how many steps before I needed to turn. I was so bone-tired that I sat on the bed and gently rocked her to get her to sleep. She projectile vomited all over me. Her father was asleep, blissfully unaware of my silent struggle.

At breaking point, I tried waking him several times in hopeless desperation before I realised I was on my own. It was just her and I. In it together.

At that moment, I let out the deepest primal sigh and unleashed all my tension with a cascade of tears. My salty overwhelm mixed with hers. I sat in the mess for a moment in complete surrender, with an inconsolable baby crying in my ear. It broke me in a way I had never experienced. I felt so out of my depth as a new mother, so consumed in the mess of mothering that I had to allow myself to be swallowed whole. The only way out of the torture was through it.

I accepted my fate, my defeat and my aloneness. My suffering was a choice and so I got back up, cleaned us both and then crawled back into bed with her side feeding. I wept as we both fell asleep. This was when I realised that no matter how much support you have, you will always have moments when you feel so alone because nothing will substitute a mother's love and service.

I'm not exaggerating when I say she screamed for the first several months of her life. Some days, the colic was from gas; other days, there was projectile vomiting from too much milk and silent reflux. I had tried everything, adjusting what I ate, how I fed, how quickly I raised her upright to burp, baby massage techniques, gripe water and a myriad of alternative natural remedies.

After months of desperate attempts, I purchased a bottle of *Infacol* from the chemist, which I was reluctant to use. I gave her a few drops under the tongue and fed her as usual. When she sat up, she did a massive burp and was quiet and content. Her father and I looked at each other with a 'WTF' look of disbelief. We were ready for the screams, but they didn't come. It was like she was a different baby. I'd love to say this relief was the new normal, but it was only short-lived. The colic eventually eased once she started crawling at 7 months.

Once my breasts settled with milk production and the colic eased, breastfeeding was a joyful experience for both of us. During my breastfeeding journey, I found it to be a beautiful, sacred experience and one to which I chose to devote my full presence.

Healing Blocked Ducts and Mastitis Naturally

My first bout of mastitis was excruciatingly painful, but I did manage to heal it naturally without antibiotics. I felt the symptoms manifest as feeling run down and feverish. I thought I had the flu, but then one breast became painfully engorged, lumpy and hot. I tried cabbage leaves in my bra and massaging my breast, but it was too painful, so I put a warm compress over the area and then immersed myself in a hot bath, deep enough to cover my breasts. After several minutes of soaking, I began massaging the infection out. A disgusting green pus squiggled out into the bath water and I roared with each motion, firmly expressing it out of my breast. This process took three days until the infection had cleared. It's one of the most intensely visceral experiences.

Some other remedies to help with milk fever are:

- Staying hydrated
- No bras or tight-fitting clothes
- Dangle feeding
- An electric toothbrush or mini vibrator can be used over the breast tissue to help break up the blocked ducts.
- Turmeric, orange and lemon hot drinks.

- Herbal tinctures.
- Frankincense or Lavender oil- diluted and massaged over the breast but not areola or nipples
- Fenugreek compress: Fill a cotton breastfeeding pad or cloth with fenugreek seeds, soak it in hot water and place the compress on the affected breast, which is held with a bra.
- Support so that you can rest.

With my second baby, I had blocked ducts and mild milk fever, though it didn't lead to infection because I knew that the underlying emotions were about doing too much, feeling resentful towards my partner at the time for not providing the support I needed. Resenting that I felt like I was the only one managing everything (giving too much) and the only one who could feed or soothe my child (there was no way I would use formula or a pacifier), so expressing the emotion helped to release the inner conflict causing the blockage so that the milk could flow again.

Having said all of this, I responded to the symptoms early and have a high pain tolerance. Whether or not you go down the natural healing route or turn towards Western medicine is a decision you will need to make based on your own body and lifestyle. Natural healing may take longer and require more rest and downtime, so if that doesn't fit your circumstances and it means taking antibiotics, then please do not entertain any shame-related beliefs because you didn't 'heal it naturally.' Your health and well-being are a personal choice and priority.

Devotional Breastfeeding

From the moment I first started breastfeeding, I had a natural desire to treat breastfeeding as a ritual to intone my milk with blessings and prayers for my growing baby. I would usually find a quiet and comfortable place to sit or lay whilst singing to my baby as she suckled from my breast. Songs and sounds would flow through me without thought. I imagined my heart radiating with love and light, passing through my breast as the milk was drawn from this space, directly from my heart and soul. Sometimes, I'd stare lovingly and think about how beautiful her life would be and how much I would pour into her to support her on her journey of self-growth and evolution. There would be times I would weep at how beautiful the experience was to nourish my child with the milk I produced for her.

This practice would call me into a deep state of devotion as a mother. During this time, I would, for the most part, remove myself from social settings to find a quiet space for us to breastfeed. I had no problem feeding in public and often did out of necessity, but this was a spiritual act of devotion that required space and presence. Not everyone understood what I was doing, but they accepted my need for quiet and privacy. If I began feeling tense or stressed, I would take a moment to breathe and ground my energy before offering my breast. I wanted my milk to flow abundantly with good energy and I continued this practice with all my children.

When I'd allow myself to open my energy to the wisdom of the grandmothers, it's as though my child was drinking nectar and ambrosia of divine consciousness flowing through my body and being filled with deep soul nutrition. Even if you decide to bottle feed, you can treat it as a ritual and brew your child's food with presence, intention and prayers.

The Cusp of Weaning

Each time you breastfeed, focus your energy and awareness towards your breasts and womb, honouring the blessings of your fertility and the many ways becoming a mother has shaped you so far. This time of transition is another rite of passage and is to be met with the same level of presence that allows you to tap into the sacredness. There are many unknown variables ahead, so you may feel the journey calling you into stillness, to connect with your yearning to feel the ripe fullness of the feminine, sharing your love with another dreamseed again or an invitation for you to gather your strength and begin the process of letting go, disconnecting from the functional act of breastfeeding.

This stage of unknowing makes weaning bittersweet because the future is uncertain. Treat this experience as if it is the last time you'll get these moments. Savour them as if you are consciously creating a memory and focus on every little detail. Breathe it all in and be with the beauty of it all, reminiscing on the first moment you brought your baby to your breast, the first moment they suckled up until now.

Cherish all the little moments of close bonding and connection, the warmth and sensations of milk flowing through your breasts to nurture your child. Allow your heart to swell with gratitude.

Weaning will usher in change as you navigate new identities outside of the breastfeeding partnership.

Conscious Weaning

The decision to wean varies from Mother to Mother. Whether it's due to a need to return to work, medical reasons, emergencies or simply the desire to regain autonomy over your body, each Mother's journey is unique. Ideally, weaning becomes an intentional ritual, transitioning into a new way of relating outside the breastfeeding relationship.

If you approach weaning as another initiation process, you can plan for it in advance, allowing for at least a week of a disrupted routine. If you have your menstrual cycle, consider dates that align with your follicular or ovulation stage, as you'll have more patience and energy to handle the challenge. The intensity of weaning can vary, but preparing for the worst and having support will help you succeed sooner. If your child shows signs of self-weaning, this process will be easier than if you feel ready, but your child is still emotionally attached.

We often underestimate children's intelligence, especially in nonverbal communication. Keep reassuring your child through your words, touch and signals so they feel safe and supported during this process, as it can be confusing for little ones. Positive association and consistency are key to an easy transition. This journey of detachment should be slow and steady, allowing your child to learn to emotionally regulate and adapt to their new identity as a big kid without feeling rejected.

Gradually and slowly wean over a few months. If you're sleep training simultaneously, this will mean not letting your child fall asleep on the breast. You would feed in a more communal space so that they begin to develop a positive association with their bedtime routine and that their bed equals sleeping alone. If they're toddlers, consider taking them out to select a new blanket, bedspread or nighttime cuddle toy to help transition them into their own bed. Make this a fun and uplifting experience so that you can help them reach this new milestone of growth and independence.

Introduce more solid foods and less breast. You may need a few diversions to distract your child's impulse to access the milk bar that is now closing. Minimise the time on the breast until you drop a feed altogether. Slowly but surely, keep eliminating breastfeeding during the day until you are breastfeeding first thing in the morning or at night. Keep one of these feeds for your deep bonding time but continue to communicate with your child what is happening to prepare for fully weaning.

Encourage their independence and tell them how proud you are and that they are growing up and turning into a big person, with a big person bed. Your calm and uplifted state will help them see this as a positive and natural step. You may need to create a link to older siblings, cousins or friends who do the same.

When you are ready to drop the last feed, you will also do this gradually by slowly limiting the time on the breast. By doing it this way, it gives your breasts a chance to dry up slowly so that you do not become engorged. If this does happen, treat it as if your milk was coming in for the first time and only express enough milk to alleviate the pressure and discomfort.

Create a simple repeatable saying for when you need to say no to your child, for instance, if you are night weaning and they keep waking to breastfeed, you can say,

> "When the sunny sun comes up, and the birds are singing, then you can have booby, ok?"

Your child may not be fully ready yet and this can be quite traumatic. You need to emotionally prepare your child to detach in the weeks leading up to weaning. Expect tantrums and protest behaviour. Let your child express their frustration and ensure they have had enough to satisfy their hunger. Offer lots of cuddles and reassurance. If you've planned for this, you will also feel committed to seeing the process through to completion and holding space for your child to express their emotions and learn this new rhythm and way of life. I waited until the cuspids- also known as eye teeth, ruptured through the gums as I offered my breasts for comfort during teething.

After emotionally preparing their children, some Mothers will go away for a weekend to create that separation and process the new identity.

Essentially, you need to prepare to wean in advance and do what works for you and your family.

Letting Go

Peppermint oil is a galactagogue and can help reduce milk supply and soothe engorgement. Blend a few drops of peppermint oil with a carrier oil and gently massage the mixture around your breast tissue, extending up to the collarbone while avoiding the nipple.

As you anoint yourself with this soothing oil blend, take a moment to bring gratitude to this intimate chapter of nurturing and connection. Reflect on the moments of closeness, the bond forged through each feeding, and the incredible gift you have given.

Connect with your wombspace, the source of life and creation and acknowledge the spectrum of emotions that may flow through your body; grief, doubt, relief and perhaps a sense of loss. Allow yourself to feel each emotion fully and understand that they are all part of this significant transition. Weaning can be bittersweet, bringing up many emotions as you regain energy and reclaim your body. It's a process of letting go and a time of renewal and self-discovery.

As you gently guide yourself through this change, honour the strength and love that have been integral to your breastfeeding journey.

Embrace the space opening up within you, both physically and emotionally and trust that this is a natural progression on your path to embodied and present Motherhood. Through this mindful ritual, find peace in the knowledge that you have provided nourishment and comfort and now, you are embracing a new phase of growth and transformation for both you and your child.

In letting go, you honour the journey and embrace new beginnings.

PART V: THE GREAT WORK
EMBRACING AND DEEPENING INTO THE LEGACY OF YOUR MOTHERHOOD

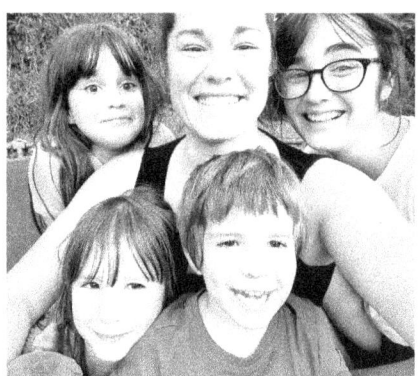

"Having kids- the responsibility of rearing good, kind, ethical human beings- is the biggest job anyone could embark on." - Maria Shiver

19

MATRESENCE
THE SACRED DANCE OF BECOMING

"The critical transition period which has been missed is matrescence, the time of mother-becoming...Giving birth does not automatically make a mother out of a woman...The amount of time it takes to become a mother needs study."
-Dana Raphael, Ph.D

Matrescence was first coined by the medical anthropologist Dana Raphael in the mid-70s. In modern-day behavioural and social science circles, Matrescence is described as the transition to motherhood associated with physiological, hormonal, social, psychological, economic, emotional, neural and cognitive changes, akin to the developmental process and transition of adolescence[1].

In my experience, this *sacred rite of passage* is the quiet unravelling and reweaving of identity. It is the awakening of new awareness in the mind, body and soul and the merging of who you were with who you are becoming. It is the bittersweet goodbye to the woman you once knew, the way she thought and moved through the world and the welcoming of the tender embrace of the mother you are now and learning to be, in all your beautiful mess.

In the stillness of the night, when you cradle your newborn, the integration from *Maiden to Mother* envelops you as you begin to understand the sacred dance between joy and exhaustion, wonder and worry, confidence and confusion as you face the often brutal truth of motherhood.

Your body, tender from birth, learns to lean in and listen, to sway to the rhythm of new life, each heartbeat a whisper of ancient wisdom, each breath a testament to the resilience of all mothers and you step forth and claim your place, and your new role.

In the early newborn days, life is a blur of monotony and chaos, of hormonal and perspective shifts, but it will lead you to discover depths of patience and courage you never knew existed. As you start to attune yourself to your new identity as a Mother and to the cacophony of needs and cries from your baby and your body, you find the voice of your inner authority. It's a gentle hum of your song that gets stronger and more confident as the days pass. This is a journey of maturation, a journey of leadership.

The expansive world you once frolicked in as a *Maiden* is now contracted around this tiny being that consumes your attention and energy. Matrescence is not merely a stage but a continual becoming, a lifelong evolution as you learn to embody your wisdom and power as a Matriarch. It is the gentle unfolding of the Mother within, a testament to the power and grace inherent in every woman. Through sleepless nights and joyous days, you emerge and transform. There can be profound grief here as you realise you are forever changed. Your mind, body and Soul will never be the same, for you have crossed the threshold into unchartered waters. It is here that you will learn to swim, channel your energy towards well-being and trust yourself to find your flow.

Integrating the Mother

If the Maiden is not honoured, integrated and allowed to gracefully step aside for the new energy to emerge through initiation, an uninitiated Mother's inner Maiden will resist her responsibilities, her call to surrender and slow down. She may throw tantrums and make reckless choices, driven by the naïve belief that she can have it all right now, leading only to depletion.

In contrast, the healthy integrated Mother understands that there is a season for everything. She embodies the wisdom of her ancestors, maturing her perspective with the patience to nurture and sow seeds over time. She delights in the magic of growth and the simple joys of living in the present. She knows that she need not sacrifice herself at the altar of motherhood unless truly called to do so.

Failing to integrate the Mother energy and embrace this balance can lead to frustration and burnout, diminishing the experience of Motherhood. This is not the path of healthy mothering, as it can result in missing out on the most precious years of a child's life, the early years when strong foundational attachments and healthy emotional bonds are formed. Children are only small for about five years, a brief but vital time where presence is the greatest investment a Mother can offer to create lasting, secure connections.

Committing to embodied mothering as the greatest work means that this role is worth more than any temporary gain from pursuing what you think you should be doing to keep up with everybody else. You cannot expect fruit from the fresh shoots of a new sapling, so you must tend to your roots. If you look at nature, those plants that bolt to seed early are under severe stress. Motherhood is an ultra-marathon, not a sprint. It requires strength, grit, resilience and humour.

It calls you to slow down, listen, respond, listen, heal, listen some more and cherish those fleeting moments of raising great human beings who will become the custodians of your legacy. The work you put in now will come back to reward you tenfold in ways that will light you up from the inside out. There will be gifts offered in seemingly mundane moments in recognition of all that you are and all that you do and have done.

The ripple effect of your service as a present and loving Mother is far greater than anything you could ever imagine. The future generations of children connected to and through your lineage and through your mothering will be thriving from a young age because of the work that you do now. This is how we heal timelines.

This is the wise way of a matriarch who nurtures the soul soil for new seeds to sprout, loving and mothering in this way becomes the ultimate gift of devotional practice.

Embodied Mothering

Embodiment is the profound experience of living fully in one's body, of being deeply connected to the physical self in a way that transcends the mundane motions of daily life. It is the art of sensing, feeling and inhabiting the body with awareness and presence. This practice brings you into intimate contact with prana, the breath, lifeforce essence and the gift of being alive.

For a new Mother, embodiment can be a healing balm that roots her into her power. After months of carrying life within, the body undergoes immense changes as suddenly, what was full is now empty and everything rearranges to accommodate a new identity and lifestyle. Motherhood can feel foreign, like an unfamiliar landscape. Embodiment invites you to reconnect with your transformed body, to inhabit it fully and to honour it for the miraculous work it has done.

Embodied mothering is about feeling each moment with acute awareness. The warmth of your baby's skin against your chest, the rhythm of breath synchronising with the heartbeat, the ache in muscles that have borne the weight of new life. The awareness of physical sensations grounds you in the present, counterbalancing the whirlwind of thoughts and emotions. To be embodied is also to embrace vulnerability. It is acknowledging the fragility of the postpartum body and mind and allowing yourself to be tender and gentle. It means listening to the body's whispers and cries and respecting its need for rest, nourishment and care.

In a society that often pushes for a rapid return to pre-pregnancy norms, embodiment is a radical act of self-compassion and acceptance. It is the practice of being here, now, in this body, with these feelings. It is about being fully alive to each moment, no matter how mundane or profound. In the sacred dance of motherhood, embodiment is a vital rhythm. It calls you to inhabit your body with reverence, honour your physical and emotional experiences and embrace the fullness of your initiation from *Maiden to Mother*.

Beyond Motherhood- The Art of Legacy Weaving

The Great Mother calls you into her deep embrace, all-consuming, evolving and expanding. She is the season of summer, wildly busy in service, though she does not lose sight of the legacy she is building. She will call for the maiden to sacrifice herself in a way that integrates energies and can uphold and regenerate her rebirth, deepening into Motherhood.

This is an initiation in and of itself, where values and priorities will be checked and refined repeatedly. Each season and cycle will bring new pains, purpose and priority. Having so many energy centres open will drain the mother; she must contain herself and stay focused on the task at hand, or she will surely burn out mentally and physically. Her passion projects may need to be shelved for a season or two as she weans off the dedicated presence that early childhood demands.

This does not mean that these dreams and passions are not pursued. They can be, of course, at the same time. However, what it does mean is that she will not be able to work feverishly towards creating and fully engaging in these pursuits that take her presence outside of the home, for it will surely lose its hearth. She will feel stretched and pulled in conflicting directions.

This is a lived torture for many creatively driven and ambitious mothers and it needs tender care to address it and find a beautiful way to walk the middle ground. The path of the devoted mother is challenging and requires a woman to surrender certain desires for the greater good.

Legacy building is a long game where the investment of time and energy has incredible long-term rewards, but these may feel so far away for a woman in the thick of the early stages of Motherhood.

Everything Has A Season

I will not be a mystery to my children, especially my daughters. I will not hide my desires or my pain as I am a fully embodied woman with hopes and dreams who also happens to be their Mother. I walk gently to emulate resilience and wild, playful curiosity to the majick and wonder of life. I plant seeds at their feet, hoping they blossom when they need colour and wonder. I share my journey honestly and as they mature, I reveal more of my edges and the beautiful mess of a woman I am so that they can sit with those parts of themselves with curiosity and humour... for they knew me from the inside and I have helped shape their world, hopefully for the better.

Poetry aside, looking at my experiences, I feel like I did everything backwards to how you were *supposed* to do life. I guess you could say that I failed to follow the rules of life. Instead, I followed my intuition and connection to a higher knowing, where I lived in a state of service, listening and responding to life and what was being asked of me. For the most part, I still live by these principles as they have helped me navigate life with a brilliant sense of wonder and resilience to view and experience life as a divine comedy and ephemeral learning journey.

I never really knew what I wanted to be. I was not someone who had a clear vision of a career. I am wildly creative and hardworking, though I was not destined to climb any hierarchical ladders or pursue status. I knew I would be a young mother and a bloody good one. I felt it in my bones, and at 21, my journey started, before I could figure out what I wanted to *be* in the world, I was just me. I fully surrendered to that journey- I lived simply and was so grateful to have had the support to stay home raising my child as a single mother in Australia. This allowed me to be fully present in raising my daughter and become curious about how I could contribute to society in a more valuable way.

When my firstborn was eighteen months old, I moved back home with my parents and began my art degree. I cried so deeply when I had to put her into childcare three days a week so I could study. Although I found the best daycare for her, it just didn't feel right, and I felt a lot of guilt. It took me three years to complete a Visual Art diploma as I could only commit to the work part-time.

THERE ARE times when I've hidden behind the excuse of motherhood in committing fully to my entrepreneurial path. The more I sit with the deeper reasoning behind it, I am met with the simple wisdom and knowing that I couldn't *'do it all'*. I couldn't stomach what was being sold to me. I know a lot of modern-day thinking tells us women that we really can have it all but the argument is moot when you consider the decimation of the village that helped to raise children. Everything has a cost. That is the law of cause and effect.

The have-it-all mentality as a blanket statement is misguided and dangerous. It hijacks the nervous system and sets women up for burnout. And what is the greater cost of all this? Build an empire- climb the corporate ladder, make bank, for what? Where are your children? How are they experiencing life? What time and energy are you investing into thriving relationships with your children? What stories will they share with you when they become adults? Will you sit with their hurt and pain or justify the neglect as your parents most likely did?

At seventeen years and four spirals deep into Mothering, I can firmly stand in my conviction and know that everything has a season. I'm not saying to give up. I'm promoting the gift of grace to oneself. What do you do when you feel like you have a bigger vision or purpose in the world beyond being a mother? Simple. Turn to the wisdom of Nature and embrace the wisdom that everything has a season.

Don't let your creativity die inside of you but don't burn the wick at both ends and die inside. Focus on your legacy instead of running the rat race. Slow down. What is meant for you will come to you. Trust yourself to stay the course. You may already be dealing with high stress or have adapted to it without realising it. Don't focus on increasing your stress levels even more (shoutout to all you neurodivergent mamas, I see you!).

The name of the game is nervous system regulation. Sometimes, it feels uncomfortable and unintuitive because we must meet all the demands of Motherhood and our budding careers. You are a powerful creatrix who can live your life by design and make better decisions. You must allocate the time to slow down and return to your centre to listen to the gentle whisper of your Soul.

When you feel like you've lost yourself, it's time to get quiet. Silence the external stimuli of the world's noise beyond what is necessary and important. Close down social media. Clear your calendar. Go sit with Nature.

Take the time you need to soften into your body and the moment, if that takes months, then it takes months. It will be worth it. You are worth it. The reclamation of your big mission and purpose is worth it but you will probably fuck it all up with distorted thinking trying to push through the chaos of your busy life. Breathe. Breathe this new 'baby' through.

Understanding your inner rhythm and approach to birthing new ideas and projects into the world is important for creating a space to immerse in your creativity and pursue a purpose beyond Motherhood. Thinking of the creative process as a birth can help you trust the process and embrace the season you are in. This shift in focus from pressure to expansion allows you to connect your creative pursuits to something larger and more profound.

In this way, you can see your vision and mission as another being, with whom you are in a dance to bring it into the world as clearly and efficiently as possible. This prepares the way for it to grow, take shape and evolve in the way it needs to, ultimately existing beyond you and hopefully providing for you in the long term.

Throughout the stages of womanhood, we witness and experience the patterns of Nature and existence, like recurrent fractals across space and time. As we gain a more comprehensive understanding of the stages and seasons of womanhood, we learn to value the interconnection of all life and the beauty found in accepting life's constantly evolving rhythms as they unfold before us.

Understanding that everything has a season reminds us to honour our inner rhythms, cultivate resilience and find solace in the ever-changing magic of life. It's a celebration of the beauty of embracing life's seasons, slowing down and being present, knowing that each chapter contributes to the rich tapestry of our human experience and adds colour and texture to our legacy as mothers.

20

THE ABYSS OF MOTHERHOOD
ILLUMINATING THE PATH THROUGH THE DARKNESS OF THE FIRST YEARS.

"The most difficult part of birth is the first year afterwards. It is the year of travail – when the soul of a woman must birth the mother inside her. The emotional labor pains of becoming a mother are far greater than the physical pangs of birth; these are the growing surges of your heart as it pushes out selfishness and fear and makes room for sacrifice and love. It is a private and silent birth of the soul, but it is no less holy than the event of childbirth, perhaps it is even more sacred."
-Joy Kusek, LCCE

Motherhood is a journey, not a destination. It will stretch you in ways beyond imagination, breaking you open to the beautiful mess of living. And you will break...oh how you will break and piece by piece, you'll build yourself up into a more mature and honest version of yourself, with each crack paving the way for a more resilient version of yourself to emerge.

Your patience and relationships will be tested, revealing any misalignments with your inner truth, the remnants of distractions from your *Maiden* self becoming more apparent and often intolerable.

There are many unknown variables to consider as you embark on your journey into what feels like an abyss. There will be days when it feels like mere survival and defeat is imminent. There might be years where you barely keep afloat, drifting aimlessly on the currents of life with no guiding rudder or winds. You'll question yourself as you develop your inner authority and intuition as a Mother. Add in all the external social and economic pressures, and you've got a melting pot bubbling with everything you need to experience an epic mental health crisis.

Nurturing the Newborn Mother

Amidst these trials, your baby will experience rapid growth and reach countless milestones in their first year. Generally speaking, just as they learn to lift their head, sit and crawl before mastering the art of walking and talking, so will you, as a new Mother, find your rhythm and groove. Give yourself lots of grace and spaciousness to figure it out. Let yourself crawl before you walk.

The more you feel seen, heard, nurtured and supported through this *sacred rite of passage*, the easier it will be for you to replenish your body and spirit, anchoring this new identity healthily.

Just as a newborn baby has needs that need to be met to thrive, so do you as a newly born Mother. We owe it to all Mothers to be able to meet more than just their basic primary needs. How we treat Mothers ripples through the field, down the line, to the future generations. We can change the world in one generation, but we can't expect Mothers to raise others when they feel like they're sinking.

Postpartum healing extends beyond nourishing foods and adequate rest. It's learning, feeling and sensing your specific needs that nourish your body, mind and Spirit.

- It's learning to nurture and soothe a dysregulated nervous system so that you can cultivate resilience.
- It's learning that your self-worth is not dependent on your productivity or performance in motherhood.
- It's unhooking from the old stories, expectations and

patriarchal conditioning of silent sacrificial labour and martyrdom.
- It's learning interdependence and allowing yourself to receive help and support, even though you know you are capable.
- It's feeling safe to surrender into the new identity and demands of motherhood whilst also surrendering to the deep receptivity of the divine feminine.
- It is allowing yourself to freely voice the power of your inner wisdom and intuition as a mother and speak up on behalf of those women in your lineage who have been silenced for generations.
- It's connecting with your creativity and expressions as a sensual woman.
- It's being part of a village and sisterhood.

This healing will become part of your living legacy as an embodied woman and Mother, but for your body to be able to access these deeper states of being you will first need to be competent in attuning and regulating your nervous system so that you come back to centre, 'calm your crazy' and create longlasting transformational change and healing.

Attuning the Nervous System

With its myriad challenges, Motherhood demands competence in understanding the intricate dance of the Autonomic Nervous System (*ANS*) and how it impacts this new way of experiencing the world. The *ANS* split into the *sympathetic* (fight or flight) and *parasympathetic* (rest and digest) systems, which govern your responses to stress and relaxation.

Postpartum stress frequently disrupts this delicate equilibrium, resulting in an overactive sympathetic system that unleashes a cascade of cortisol. This imbalance casts a shadow over a mother's health and her initiation into Motherhood. Recognising signs of dysregulation and addressing them early is essential for restoring homeostasis.

Nervous system dysregulation intensifies the body's stress response, activating the *hypothalamic-pituitary-adrenal axis (HPA)* and elevates cortisol levels. This surge contributes to feelings of anxiety, tension and overwhelm, disrupting emotional regulation and sleep-wake cycles, leading to overstimulation, insomnia and burnout. It also upsets the balance of mood-regulating neurotransmitters like serotonin and dopamine, impairing cognitive functions such as memory, concentration and decision-making.

The term *'tired and wired'* aptly describes the simultaneous fatigue and mental overstimulation that new mothers often experience. This state arises from a confluence of sleep deprivation, hormonal fluctuations and the continuous demands of caring for a newborn.

The physical exhaustion from lack of sleep and the mental stress of new motherhood create a hyperalert state, making relaxation elusive and intensifying feelings of overwhelm and anxiety. Strategies to promote restorative sleep, relaxation and stress management are crucial during this period and it is vital that you rest after giving birth.

THE VAGUS NERVE, a vital component of the parasympathetic nervous system, plays a key role in regulating the body's stress responses and maintaining balance during the postpartum period.

Extending from the brainstem to the abdomen, the vagus nerve influences heart rate, digestion and immune response. Its activation fosters calm and relaxation, counterbalancing the sympathetic nervous system's 'fight or flight' reactions. For new mothers, stimulating the vagus nerve can help mitigate the physiological impacts of postpartum stress, such as elevated cortisol levels and disrupted sleep patterns.

By attuning to these signals, new mothers can navigate the complexities of postpartum life with greater resilience and well-being. Through self-awareness and proactive self-care, it is possible to transition from merely surviving to truly thriving in motherhood.

Identifying and addressing dysregulation requires time to learn, but it is a crucial path towards healthy embodied leadership as a present and loving parent. It also gives you the tools to co-regulate with your children and role model necessary life skills.

. . .

Techniques for Regulation

- **Breathing Exercises:** Simple practices like deep belly breathing can activate the parasympathetic nervous system, promoting relaxation. Breathing in for a count of four, holding for four and exhaling for six is a technique that is easy to practice. Just remember to make you exhale longer.
- **Gentle Movement:** Activities like yoga, tai chi, freestyle dance or even gentle stretching can help regulate the nervous system by releasing built-up tension and promoting physical relaxation.
- **Sensory Soothing:** Engaging the senses through soothing music, aromatherapy or gentle touch can help calm the nervous system. A warm bath with Epsom salts, listening to nature sounds and massaging with calming oils can provide sensory relief. Sometimes, a change of environment is needed for you and your baby. Wearing *'Loop Earplugs'* can also help with sensory overstimulation, such as dealing with high-pitched crying.
- **Bilateral Stimulation (BLS):** Using alternating sensations, such as tapping or pulsing, BLS can help to activate the parasympathetic nervous system by engaging both hemispheres in the brain. A common practice in EMDR therapy is called the *'Butterfly Hug'* and can help to create a sense of calm.
- **Staying hydrated and nourished:** Staying hydrated and eating throughout the day is important to balance your energy. Eat within an hour of waking to avoid a cortisol spike. Be mindful of caffeine dependence, especially if you experience anxiety.
- **Grounding Techniques:** Grounding exercises, such as walking barefoot on grass, holding a cold object or focusing on physical sensations, can help anchor you in the present moment and regulate the nervous system. Gentle self-massage and 'brushing' can also help with sensory dysregulation.

- **Stimming:** Self-stimulatory behaviour, known as 'stimming', is the repetition of physical movement, sounds, words or objects to soothe and settle emotions and stress and regulate the nervous system.
- **Singing, chanting or humming:** Helps to stimulate the vagus nerve and is shown to stimulate the release of endorphins, the body's natural feel-good chemicals, which can enhance your mood and reduce feelings of sadness or depression commonly experienced during the postpartum period.
- **Establish Boundaries:** Set realistic expectations for yourself and communicate your needs to your partner, family and friends. It's okay to ask for help and to delegate tasks when needed. Establishing boundaries around your time and energy can help prevent feelings of overwhelm.
- **Express Yourself:** Find healthy ways to express your thoughts and emotions. Whether through journaling, creative expression or talking with a trusted friend or therapist, expressing yourself can help release pent-up emotions and promote emotional well-being. For some neurodivergent mothers, verbal processing is a form of stimming.
- **Connect with Others:** Stay connected with friends, family and other new mothers for emotional support and companionship. Joining a local women's circle, support group, or online community can provide a sense of belonging, validation and opportunities to share experiences and resources.

Mental Health Awareness for New Mothers

In the delicate journey of postpartum and learning to adapt to your new identity and rhythms of life, it's crucial to heed the silent alarms that signal potential risks to mental health, beyond the very normal fluctuations of nervous system responses to mothering. While the postpartum period is filled with joy and wonder, it can also be fraught with stressors that impact your well-being. Sometimes, in the blur of daily life, you may not realise you aren't coping, so talk to your trusted family and friends so that they can keep an eye on your mental health and understand the warning signs to empower you to seek support and navigate this transformative journey with resilience.

Silent Alarms

- Pay attention to fluctuations in mood, from intense happiness to overwhelming sadness, anger or irritability. While mood swings are common in the postpartum period, persistent feelings of sadness, hopelessness or anxiety may indicate a more serious issue such as postpartum depression, anxiety or PTSD.
- Disrupted sleep is a hallmark of early motherhood, but severe insomnia or excessive sleepiness could be red flags for underlying mental health concerns. Difficulty falling or staying asleep, even when the baby rests warrants attention.
- Changes in appetite, whether excessive or diminished, can be indicative of mental health challenges. Pay attention to significant weight loss or gain and changes in eating patterns or food preferences.
- Physical symptoms such as headaches, digestive issues or unexplained aches and pains may accompany mental health disorders. These symptoms should not be ignored, especially if they persist despite medical evaluation.
- New mothers often experience shifts in socialisation due to the demands of caring for a newborn. However, isolating oneself from friends and family or withdrawing from previously enjoyed activities may signal deeper emotional struggles.
- *Dorsal Vagal Shutdown* occurs when the nervous system perceives a threat as overwhelming or inescapable, leading to a shutdown or *'freeze'* response. Look for behaviour characterised by immobilisation, dissociation, and feeling stuck, checked out, numb or disconnected from oneself or your surroundings.

- While fleeting thoughts of harm or accidents are common in new parents, persistent and distressing intrusive thoughts may be a sign of mental health conditions.
- In rare but severe cases, postpartum psychosis can develop rapidly, usually within the first two weeks after childbirth. Watch for symptoms such as hyper-arousal, increased physical and emotional tension, confusion, hallucinations, delusions, extreme mood swings and paranoia. If you or someone you know experiences these symptoms, seek immediate medical attention, as postpartum psychosis is a medical emergency.

By recognising these silent alarms and taking proactive steps to address them, you can prioritise your mental health and well-being, paving the way for a more fulfilling and joyful motherhood experience. If you or someone you know experiences any of the above, it's essential to reach out for support without shame. Do not suffer in silence. Early intervention can be lifesaving. Talk to a healthcare provider, therapist or trusted loved one about your concerns.

Normalise seeking help and remember it is a sign of strength. Though you may have moments, you are not alone on this journey.

Neuroplasticity- Repatterning the Brain

In the context of postpartum mental health and nervous system regulation, the phrase "neurons that fire together wire together" refers to the concept of neuroplasticity, which is the brain's ability to adapt and change in response to experiences. When neurons in the brain are activated together repeatedly, they strengthen their connections, making it more likely for them to fire together in the future.

In postpartum mental health, this concept underscores the importance of engaging in positive, adaptive behaviours and thought patterns to strengthen neural circuits associated with emotional regulation, resilience and well-being. Eliminate unhealthy behaviours and distractions. Be mindful of what you consume and question whether the input is food for the soul or 'junk' food. Think of it like going to a psychological gym, where you focus on strengthening the 'weaker' side to bring everything into balance. It can take time to build new muscle, so be curious and playful in your approach so that you continue to actively participate in creating the changes that bring you into desired states of well-being.

∽

My Journey Through Dark Abyss

With a brain that seeks novelty, it was a special kind of hell to live in a simple, monotonous, baby-led routine. It felt like the same shit, different day and it was in those newborn days as a walking milk machine that I started to feel like I was losing myself.

The identity shift from *Maiden to Mother* was relatively easy for me. My life was simple. I lived in a rainforest shack and was completely enthralled and present with my daughter. Life slowed right down, but I was ready for it. My relationship did not last the first year; all of the cracks showed up like deep, irreparable crevices and I knew that I had to be the one to free us all from moving through the motions of pretending to be a happy family when we both knew we were not suited as longterm partners despite my yearning for that type of connection. We were both young and naive and even though we split, we remained friends and co-parents.

Six years and another baby later, my mental health was impacted by a psychologically abusive marriage, in which I had to gather the strength to leave before the first year, carrying guilt and shame for breaking up another family. It was one of the hardest decisions I've ever had to make, but one I am so grateful to have trusted my intuition despite the backlash and abuse I received from those who weren't privy to what happened behind closed doors.

I never really understood the intensity and torture of sleep deprivation until my third daughter was born. My first two slept through the night. They had a natural rhythm and sleep deprivation was only linked to the newborn weeks. So, entering into my 3rd spiral of mothering, I was pretty confident, perhaps even arrogant.

I was in my early 30's and felt like a seasoned pro, but my little Aquarian wild card snapped me out of my complacency. After all that I had been through in the past, she broke me, and after having walked through that darkness, I am grateful for what I learned.

My little 'Squish' was a cutie, but she didn't like sleeping. I felt like I tried all the tricks and she would only sleep for an hour at a time. The newborn season was pretty easy, but the following 3 years were hell! My life consisted of constantly interrupted sleep and running on empty. I felt like there were days I was running on fumes. It's not her fault by any means, she was my super sensitive velcro baby and I was not supported by my partner, who was in active alcohol addiction at the time.

I felt extremely isolated and alone. There is a reason sleep deprivation is used as a form of torture, as it is an assault on the soul and, over time, annihilates your ability to think rationally. I was bone-tired and burnt out. My mental health suffered and there were times when suicidal ideation crept in. I didn't want to kill myself. I loved my life. I just wanted the pain to end. I had to fight off intrusive thoughts constantly. The pain was exasperated by the fact that I was alone in it all, walking the floor with a baby that wouldn't settle.

Back then, I thought I was responsible for protecting my partner's sleep because he was up early and worked with heavy machinery as the sole income provider. I felt like we couldn't afford him to be tired, so I sacrificed myself at the altar of motherhood. I never really asked for help, I was a 'strong woman' and consequentially spiralled into adrenal shutdown, which took years to recover from. It's why I advocate for asking for help and seeking support from the village- because, for the most part- I didn't think I had any of that and suffered immensely.

I knew I was suffering and I kept quiet. I was angry and knew my thinking was distorted, so I didn't tell anyone. I forged on trusting the strength of my mental fortitude to get me through. I have a very strong mind and know my limits, so I continued trudging along. The phrase "This too shall pass" helped me claw my way back to reality when I kept slipping into the dark abyss of motherhood.

I don't share this to scare you. I share this because it is a stark reality that many women face. Some of you won't be able to afford or access therapy and so this is when you'll need to summon the strength of your ancestors to get you through those dark nights of the soul.

There might be times when you feel run down, feeling so completely overwhelmed and touched out that you will need to break, so break, emotionally.

Let yourself shatter and trust that you'll pick yourself back up after the fallout. I've learned that sometimes we need to shatter to rearrange the pieces of ourselves that reflect the mother we need to be. We are still learning. I can't even count how many times I've hidden in the bathroom, ugly-crying, completely shattered. And maybe it's because I'm a water sign, but those deep guttural cries cleanse the soul and clear up space. It's like emptying the cache on your computer browser so it can run more optimally!

There may be times when you'll feel like you're coasting through life, where everything feels like it's coming at you at once, where you feel like you're treading water and getting nowhere. You may feel like you used to be able to juggle 10 balls at once, and now you can only keep 2 up in the air. This is ok. Your journey might be learning to be with what is- not what you think should be.

If you prioritise your vitality, you'll recover sooner. Just because you can only keep 2 balls in the air right now, doesn't mean you've lost the ability to juggle 10. If your nervous system completely shuts down, you won't be able to juggle at all. Then what?

The only way out of the darkness is through it. Simplicity is key and for the most part, I've found that adopting the perspective of this being another initiation or birth, will help you anchor to something bigger that's being birthed through you, calling you to restore your power as a creator.

When I felt like I had lost my way, I would joke that I'd taken the scenic route. It does feel like I've bush-bashed my way through most of my life. Archetypally, I've always been the type of person who finds a new route. A pathfinder and way-shower. But just because I can make carrying the load uphill look easy doesn't mean it isn't heavy. Just because it looks like I know where I'm going doesn't mean that I do. It means I've learned to listen and be present with life as it moves through me, figuring it out along the way. It doesn't mean I don't want to drop everything and run away from my responsibilities, because some days I do, but I won't because I am deeply rooted.

I have learnt to lean in and listen to the greater wisdom at play. When I'm feeling lost, I have to take a moment to catch my breath, take a radically honest look at my life and adjust to the greater dream I have been gifted, which aligns me to a path congruent with my legacy as a matriarch.

Sometimes, you think you're walking in circles when it's actually a spiral. Sometimes, you take the scenic route in life, look back and laugh because you realise you were too proud to stop and ask for directions!

So, how do you get back on the path and move forward when you feel like you're walking in the dark? Firstly, it is important to take a look around and accept where you are now. It's not where you want to be, so map this space (your thoughts, feelings and behaviours) so that in future, you will know the language and scenery of this space and you won't lose yourself in it.

To take a step forward you need to set realistic expectations, recognising that the postpartum period is a time of adjustment and transition. Be with what is, not the fantasy you created before your baby came earthside. You may have been an over-achiever and over-functioning in all areas of your life and then suddenly feel like a useless blob compared to what you're used to. The initiation into motherhood can be humbling and requires humility. Remember, you have completely changed from the inside out.

Find the humour in your perceived failings. So you had a bad day? Did you walk outside with your pants on back to front? Forgot to put your top back up after breastfeeding, and you've walked around with your tit hanging out? Did your baby have a 'poosplosion' blowout and there's pumpkin soup shit up their back to their neck and you're in the middle of grocery shopping? Did they vomit all through the car and all their spare clothes, so you have to wrap them in your shirt and drive home in your bra and knickers? Did you climb into your baby's cot to settle them but break the slats? Did your toddler derobe themselves in the middle of a busy supermarket because you've raised little wildlings and clothes are too restricting? Are you a blubbering mess, like you're not ok but you know you're ok, so you end up laughing while you're crying and end up looking like an unhinged maniac? Great! You're human. (This all happened to me, by the way)

See if you can find the humour in your human experience. It makes life a wonderful divine comedy and I promise it makes everything easier to deal with. You can be a beautiful human, a glorious mess and a fantastic Mother.

You'll need to figure out how you can support your vitality simply. This is the main focus on returning home to yourself after your identity has shifted. Think nutrition, hydration, mental, emotional and spiritual health. Simplify things so that you can have easy wins.

This will help build motivation and momentum. How can you be more 'selfish' to get your needs met? I say this because many women are natural givers and nurturers to the point of depletion and then they feel bad for taking time or resources to nourish themselves. This needs to change.

Reality Checks

When you have negative thoughts and distorted thinking, I would recommend sounding all of that out to trusted friends, family or a therapist to help lift the weight of the gloom. Only talk to those that will hold a safe space for you to share.

It is so easy to spiral into a lack mentality, black-and-white thinking and absolutes when you are completely depleted. Survival mode limits your capacity for creative and optimistic thinking. During the torturous years of my severe sleep deprivation, I didn't trust myself with my thoughts or what I was seeing. There were days when I was seeing things, not quite hallucinations, but it was as if there was a lag in my perception, so my brain would fill in the blanks based on my inner narrative which wasn't good. This is important to know because it can affect your intimate relationships.

Having a support network to *'reality check'* you during these dark times can gently challenge irrational thoughts or fears, provide a more balanced perspective and help reframe situations in a more positive light, helping you to look for opportunities and positive outcomes instead.

Reality checks during early motherhood can provide validation and perspective, helping you feel understood and reminding you that you are not alone. Emotional support from friends and family offers comfort, reassurance and a listening ear, making it easier to manage difficult emotions. They can also provide practical assistance with tasks like childcare and household chores, reducing stress and allowing you to focus on self-care and bonding with your baby.

It's also important to note that every mother's experience of motherhood is unique, and there is no one-size-fits-all approach to navigating the challenges that come with it. No matter how many books you've read, honouring your journey and trusting your instincts as you find what works best for you and your baby is essential.

Writing this chapter has allowed me to reflect upon all of my postpartum journeys and think about the insights and wisdom that would be the most valuable as you navigate the first few years of motherhood. Here they are:

- Motherhood can be messy, unpredictable and full of ups and downs. It's important to remember that you don't have to be perfect and making mistakes along the way is okay. That's how we learn and grow.
- Focus on progress, learning and growth rather than striving for perfection. Attuned and embodied motherhood is not something you can master from reading all the books, you have to put it into action and adapt to your circumstances.
- "This too shall pass" is a simple phrase that will help you remember that the moments you feel completely consumed and out of your depth are only temporary.
- Rather than getting overwhelmed by thinking too far ahead, focus on taking each day as it comes. Simplify your life. Break tasks down into smaller, manageable steps and celebrate your victories, no matter how small they may seem. If you're

neurodivergent, use ChatGPT or GoblinTools to help with task management. It will help with the mental load.
- While motherhood certainly comes with its challenges, it's also filled with moments of joy, wonder and love. Take time to celebrate and savour these moments, no matter how small they seem.
- Laugh at yourself. Try not to take life too seriously.
- You are enough just as you are and are doing the best that you can for your baby. When you know better, you do better. Trust in your abilities as a mother and remember that you deserve love, support and self-compassion.
- You know your baby better than anyone else, so trust your instincts and intuition when caring for them. You are uniquely qualified to meet your baby's needs, even if it doesn't always feel that way.
- You don't have to do it all alone. It's okay to ask for help from your partner, family, friends or healthcare providers when needed. Seeking support doesn't make you weak, it makes you human.
- Self-care is not selfish, it's essential. Make time to prioritise your physical, emotional and mental well-being, even if it's just for a few minutes each day. Remember that you can't pour from an empty cup, so caring for yourself is crucial for caring for your baby.
- Motherhood is full of ups and downs. It's normal to feel overwhelmed, exhausted or unsure sometimes. Just because you only see the highlight reel of other mums doesn't mean they don't experience the same ups and downs. Most people are masters at masking in public. Permit yourself to feel whatever you're feeling and know it's okay to ask for help when needed.
- Surround yourself with a supportive sisterhood of women who lift you up and cheer you on. Whether it's other new mums, online communities or a local women's circle, having a tribe of women who understand what you're going through can make a difference.

- The first year of your baby's life will fly by faster than you can imagine, so cherish every moment, even the challenging ones. Take time to savour the little things, like cuddles, smiles and milestones, because before you know it, they'll be all grown up. You will never get this time back, so consider what that goal/career move/ project is going to cost you.
- While the first year of motherhood can be incredibly challenging, it also gets easier over time. As you and your baby settle into a routine and you gain confidence as a mother, things will feel more manageable.
- Remember that you are doing a great job as a Mother, even when it doesn't feel like it. Your love, care and presence are the most important things you can give your baby; you're already doing an amazing job just by being there for them. You're hard on yourself because you care so much.
- Your relationship with your partner will be radically tested in the first year. Make time to connect and reality-check each other. Focus on the wins you have together. Remember, they are also navigating a new identity.

ABOVE ALL, be kind and gentle with yourself. Give yourself grace as you navigate the beautifully messy unfurling of motherhood. You've got this and you are not alone. Find or create a sisterhood that uplifts, encourages and supports you with friendship and humour, share resources and emotional support and remember it takes a village to raise a child and new mother.

21

REPARENTING YOURSELF
HEAL YOUR INNER CHILD AND BREAK CYCLES

"You can't go back and change the beginning, but you can start where you are and change the ending."
- C.S. Lewis

Reparenting yourself as you step into motherhood is a journey of self-discovery, healing and empowerment. It's about embracing the opportunity to nurture and care for your inner child with love, compassion and intentionality while cultivating self-awareness, self-compassion and self-care practices that support your emotional well-being and resilience as you mother your child. The journey forward is recognising the need to mature from a young Maiden's thoughts, beliefs and behaviours into that of a grounded, mature and responsible Mother. Reparenting yourself allows maturation to gift you a renewed sense of identity and freedom in your new evolved state of being.

This process acknowledges the impact of your upbringing and parental relationships on your identity, beliefs and behaviours. It empowers you to consciously parent yourself with the kindness, empathy and understanding that you would offer to a child in need. It's about embracing the opportunity to heal old wounds, break free from negative patterns and create a vision of Motherhood that reflects your values, priorities and aspirations, setting healthy boundaries, cultivating compassionate self-talk and embodying the type of Mother you want to be. It's about prioritising your well-being, honouring your needs and desires and creating a nurturing and supportive environment for yourself and your children. By embracing this journey of self-discovery and growth, you can step into motherhood with confidence, grace and a profound sense of inner peace.

Trauma and Adverse Childhood Experiences

To move forward in life consciously, sometimes you need to step back, dip your toes into the past and figure out what worked well and what didn't so that you can do your best to heal from the wounds of the past and avoid projecting your unresolved trauma onto your children and repeating familiar cycles. A starting point is to take the *Adverse Childhood Experiences (ACE)* quiz online, which looks at trauma and adverse childhood experiences. These are:

- Physical, sexual, and emotional abuse.
- Emotional and physical neglect.
- Living with a family member with mental health or substance use disorders.
- Witnessing domestic violence.
- Sudden separation from a loved one.
- Poverty.
- Racism and discrimination.
- Violence in the community.

CHILDREN with a high *ACE* score are more likely to be disadvantaged in adulthood due to the increased risk of experiencing mental health issues, substance abuse problems and chronic diseases, among other challenges.

When you're ready, take some time to reflect on your childhood and the parenting you received. Detach from any emotions and stories that arise and objectively examine your parents' actions from your adult perspective. Try to understand their behaviour by walking a mile in their shoes. This exercise is about collecting data to heal from the past and leverage it into becoming a healthy, present and loving Mother.

As you canvas your past to paint your future, ask reflective questions to uncover patterns and gain a deeper understanding. Consider the environment you grew up in, the presence of stressors, experiences of abuse or addiction, the safety and security of your home and your parents' strengths and shortcomings.

Reflect on the lessons learned from your childhood, what needs were met or unmet and what you would change if given the chance. As you delve into this inquiry, you may gain insights into your parents' experiences and how they influenced their parenting style. It doesn't excuse or justify unhealthy behaviour, but it can clarify your parenting aspirations.

To go deeper on this exploration, you would examine your parents' upbringing or ask them similar questions to uncover ancestral patterns that shape your family. By recognising patterns of behaviour, fostering self-compassion and seeking out support specific to your needs, you can begin to address and heal the wounds from your past. Setting healthy boundaries, building resilience and cultivating coping strategies are key aspects of this process and will help you in life and Motherhood.

Gentle Parenting

Gentle parenting focuses on empathy, positive discipline, connection and communication. Instead of reacting with anger, parents seek to understand their child's emotions and developmental needs. They use guidance and logical consequences, avoiding punishment and coercive control. This approach builds trust and mutual respect, leading to strong parent-child relationships. Gentle parenting acknowledges the child as sovereign with their unique thoughts, feelings and needs and seeks to foster a strong and secure attachment between parent and child.

The benefits include promoting positive behaviour, building and strengthening emotional intelligence and resilience, encouraging healthy interdependence, boosting self-esteem, engaging in respectful communication and breaking harmful parenting patterns.

Part of the process of reparenting yourself may involve this gentle parenting approach, which may feel foreign, especially for Gen X and elder millennials as the style of parenting from the late 1970s to early 1990s is vastly different from today as we now have more information and resources that are readily available thanks to the internet. Verbal, emotional and physical abuse coupled with neglect and disconnect were considered normal 'back in the day' which created a generation of hypervigilant and independent children who are now unlearning these behaviours and discovering ways to regulate their nervous systems whilst parenting their own children.

Here's how gentle reparenting can unfold in practice:

1. Take time to connect with your inner child through practices such as meditation, visualisation or inner child work. Tune into the emotions, memories and needs that arise and offer yourself the love, comfort and support that your inner child craves. This work includes your inner teenage years as part of integrating your *Maiden*. Be the parent that you needed back then.
2. Prioritise self-care practices that nourish your body, mind and spirit and regulate your nervous system through activities such as; mindfulness, yoga, journaling, music, dance, somatic therapy, making fun memories or spending time in nature. By tending to your well-being, you will model self-love and respect to your children and create a foundation of resilience and vitality that you can build on.

3. Practice setting healthy boundaries to honour your needs and protect your energy as you navigate the demands of Motherhood. Communicate your boundaries clearly and assertively and prioritise activities and relationships that align with your core values and support your overall well-being.
4. Pay attention to your internal dialogue and practice replacing self-criticism and judgment with kindness and encouragement. Remember, words are spells, so choose them wisely. The way that you speak to yourself matters. Offer yourself words of affirmation, reassurance, forgiveness and support. Treat yourself with the same gentleness and compassion that you would to your own child during challenging times. You deserve that!
5. Embrace Neurodivergence. This refers to natural variations in brain functioning, including conditions such as autism, ADHD, dyslexia, and more. In the past, neurodivergent individuals may have been undiagnosed, misunderstood, stigmatised or pathologised, leading to feelings of shame or inadequacy. Honouring neurodivergence involves advocating for your own needs, cultivating safe spaces and friendships to unmask, managing stimulatory needs, creating healthy boundaries, sharing your story, seeking out resources, support groups and communities that celebrate neurodiversity and provide validation and affirmation. It also involves fostering an inclusive and accepting environment at home, where differences are celebrated as a natural and beautiful aspect of human variation and accommodated rather than suppressed or judged.
6. Envision the type of mother you want to be and the kind of family life you want to create. Allow yourself to draw upon inspiration from mothers around you, dream big and imagine a future filled with love, joy and connection. Use this vision as a guiding light to inspire and motivate you on your journey of reparenting and self-discovery. Come back to your vision or create a new one as you journey through life, as it may evolve

or priorities may change over time, especially if you decide to grow your family.

GENTLY REPARENTING yourself as you transition into Motherhood can create a foundation of healing, self-compassion and empowerment, guiding you toward becoming the Mother you aspire to be. This journey is not always easy, but it is enriching, offering continuous opportunities for growth, transformation and profound connection with yourself and your children. This is where true change begins.

Cycle Breaking

The journey of maturing from a Maiden into a Mother is to develop your ability to respond to life rather than react. This takes practice. When you master this, you will find the joy of being a Mother, the calm amongst the chaos and the beauty in the mess. Responsibilities are not burdens but rather an invitation towards embodying your power and duty as a leader.

It is said that pain moves down the family line until someone is brave and willing to feel and heal it. Cycle breaking is magnanimous work. It can be exhausting and is ever so rewarding, for the work that you do now will liberate the children in your lineage, perhaps the most important work you can do as a matriarch, and it is so often invisible.

It happens in the moments where you catch yourself reacting when your mind is consumed and animated with stories from the past, obsessing over things beyond your control and rather than engage in patterns of unhealthy learned behaviour and coping strategies, you take a breath, regulate yourself and respond in a way that is suitable and practical for the situation at play. This is powerful incremental work.

There's an age-old adage of 'wait until you have a child that is just like you' as if to insinuate how terrible you were. But if you are lucky enough to have a child similar to you, you'll soon realise how easy it is to love you.

There is a deep healing that takes place as a parent when you see reflections of your own self expressed in your children, when you have the realisation of how young you were and begin to grasp the scope of experiences you've had in your lifetime and any trauma associated with them.

Being a responsible adult caretaker can be triggering on so many levels, so learning to reparent yourself will give you the tools you need to move through life with emotional resilience and embodied wisdom. It will ground you to a deeper presence of purpose and help you to ebb and flow with the chaos that children can bring with them and in doing so you will find the stillness within to hold your own during times of stress so that your wounds do not bleed onto your children. You stop projecting the trauma from the past into their future and stand as a powerful cycle breaker and guardian of future generations, proudly stating,

"This ends with me!"

Healing your Inner Child

Healing and integrating your inner child involves a three-level approach focusing on the mind, body and soul. Somatic exercises, body-based therapies and psychological techniques are effective in releasing stored tension, trauma, repressed emotion and memory trapped in the body or subconscious mind. Some of the most effective modalities are as follows;

- Somatic Experiencing (SE), developed by Dr. Peter Levine, helps release trauma from the body through gentle exercises and awareness.
- Internal Family Systems (IFS) therapy views the mind as consisting of various parts. Through guided visualisation, dialogue and compassionate inquiry, individuals can establish a relationship with these parts, offering them understanding, acceptance and healing to those parts carrying childhood wounds.
- Eye Movement Desensitization and Reprocessing (EMDR) is another powerful therapy that helps process traumatic memories through bilateral stimulation, fostering healing and integration.

- Wombwork explores and heals energetic and emotional imprints in the womb, complementing other healing practices. By reconnecting with the wisdom of the womb and addressing any unresolved issues related to birth, conception, or early childhood experiences, individuals can cultivate a deeper sense of self-awareness, healing and empowerment.
- Breathwork regulates the nervous system and trauma-informed movement practices facilitate self-expression and release at the root.
- Somatic Practices such as bodywork, craniosacral, network spinal analysis and spinal flow techniques, tai-chi, yoga, acupuncture, shiatsu, dance and pulsing are powerful body-led practices that bring awareness to tension stored in the body and help to optimise the function of the nervous system to self-regulate and release stressors more effectively.
- Creative expression and nature connection provide nonverbal outlets for processing childhood wounds and fostering empowerment.

Envisioning the Mother You Want to Become

Take a moment to reflect deeply upon everything you've read so far. You are the world for your child and are responsible for the initial imprinting baby receives in the womb and the formative years of development. How you mother will directly shape your child's consciousness and how they experience life. It will impact their sense of belonging, identity, self-image, inner critic, creativity and relationships. I believe that the most impactful work in this world is that of a Mother.

As you step into this role, it's natural to reflect on your upbringing, what worked, what didn't and what you aspire to recreate or change moving forward. Envisioning the mother you want to become is a powerful and positive exploration that empowers you to be present, intentional and aligned with your deepest values and aspirations. This process is not about dwelling on past mistakes or trauma, it's about rewriting the scripts of your childhood and crafting a new story for your family, embracing the limitless potential of the present moment and the boundless possibilities of the future.

THE BEAUTY in this is that you can revisit this process as you deepen into the season of Motherhood, for as you know better, you do better.

Mapping Motherhood

One of the best ways to anchor your vision of Motherhood is to write out what you value and the qualities that inspire you and journal your thoughts and feelings around them to create a map. Remember, the map is not the territory, but it can help you navigate the undefined landscapes of your motherhood journey and align your beliefs and behaviours around your desires.

Look at the values list in the Notes section at the end of this book and intuitively select twenty that resonate. Once you have that list, narrow it down again to your top three to five values. Put some thought into your values as some can overlay or are implied in each other, like trust, integrity, honesty and transparency. If you find this task a challenge, think about mother figures who inspire you and what values they embody.

Journalling Prompts

- How do/will I embody my core values as a Mother?
- What are my desires in life as a mother and beyond that role?
- What beliefs do I need to have to embody the Mother I want to become?
- What changes can I make now?
- How would this version of myself be expressed? (how does she think, behave, act, create etc.)
- What drives me, and what makes me happy?
- What type of world do I want my children to live in?

- What type of world do I want seven generations forward to experience?
- What are the qualities of this world I want to experience with my children? (this will help you to establish a legacy)
- If there were NO RESTRICTIONS or limitations, what would I do/create in the world as a Mother?
- What can I do to support and regulate my nervous system?
- How do I want to be remembered?
- What type of community/village do I want to create or be a part of?
- Why is this important to me?
- What does my ideal family life look like?
- How will I know that I've achieved this?
- How will I acknowledge and celebrate my success as a Mother?
- How can I support and forgive myself for my mistakes?
- Who can I ask for support or help?
- In what ways would I sabotage myself?
- What story/belief would that validate? (I'm a terrible Mother/not good enough)
- What triggers do I have from childhood, and how can I support myself when they are being activated- so that I can come back into alignment with who I want to be
- What beliefs does this version of myself have?
- How can I let go of these beliefs?
- What are some new beliefs that hold me to a higher standard as a present and loving Mother?

Mother Journey

The following is a guided journey to bring life to your vision and version of Motherhood. Read through the script to get an idea of what to do, or record it as a voice note and use it as a guided meditation that you can listen to with headphones.

. . .

To BEGIN YOUR JOURNEY, find a space to relax and disconnect from the outside world. You may like to light a candle on your birth altar and surround yourself with items that inspire your desired expressions of the Mother you choose to be.

> *Close your eyes and take a few slow, deep breaths, guiding your breath down into your womb. Feel your belly rise and fall with your breath, allowing yourself to become fully present in the moment. Notice what you notice. As you exhale, bring some gentle movement into your body, relaxing your jaw, tongue and shoulders. Allow yourself permission to release any lingering tension or doubt. Continue to breathe deeply and rhythmically and allow yourself to open up to the vision of the Mother you want to become.*

> *Stay with this breath until you feel connected to your vision and fully present and grounded in your body. Imagine vividly embodying the qualities and characteristics most important to you as a Mother. Visualise or feel the way you interact with your child.*

> *See yourself creating a nurturing and supportive environment where your child feels safe, valued and empowered to express themselves fully. Visualise the values and beliefs you want to instil in your child and how you embody and exude those through your own actions and behaviours. Picture yourself breathing life into your child while prioritising your self-care and emotional well-being, modelling healthy communication and boundaries. See yourself building a relationship built on trust, respect, creativity and acceptance.*

> *As you immerse yourself in this vision, see what else comes through intuitively and pay attention to any feelings or insights that may arise. Notice what you notice. Pay atten-*

tion to how you feel in your body and move with the energy as it flows through you.

Journey through the timeline of your child's life and the energy you want to create around this and see yourself growing and thriving with your child, honouring their divine purpose by celebrating milestones and rites of passage with them.

Paint a picture of forgiveness around yourself when you feel like you've stuffed up along the way.

When you've finished, come back into the present moment and reflect upon what came through for you.

ONCE YOU HAVE CRYSTALISED your vision, consider what practical steps you can take to align your actions and behaviours. Reflect upon the lessons learned from your childhood, both positive and negative and identify what you want to carry forward and what you want to leave behind.

22

REVIVAL OF THE VILLAGE
DE-URBANISING MOTHERHOOD AND REKINDLING RESILIENCE

"Mothers really were not built to raise babies not only by themselves, but with only a partner. For millions of years, a woman had much more than just her husband to help rear her young… This whole idea of 'it takes a village to raise a child' is exactly how we're supposed to live."

-Helen Fisher

In today's fast-paced world, many mothers find themselves navigating the profound changes of pregnancy and motherhood largely alone. Extended families are often scattered across different cities or even countries and the demands of work and other responsibilities leave little time for fostering deep connections within communities, let alone oneself.

Social media, while offering a semblance of connection, often exacerbates feelings of isolation and inadequacy as mothers compare themselves to curated images of perfection. The 'highlight reel' seems to highlight your perceived failure and inadequacy and the squeaky clean commercials juxtapose against your messy mothering, subscribe you to the belief that miracle products are the remedy and cure to your burnout. I don't know about you, but I greatly advocate simple prevention over complex cures.

Moreover, the emphasis on individualism has led to a culture of hypervigilant, overstimulated and over-functioning adults where asking for help is seen as a sign of weakness rather than a natural part of the human experience. As a result, new mothers may feel reluctant to seek support, leading to feelings of shame, loneliness, dread, anxiety, postpartum depression or even psychosis.

If you look at the career climb of men, you can see that the ladder of success is built upon the backs of women who, often without a choice in the matter, are expected to be the primary caregivers of children. Under the structure of the industrialised nuclear family, men went to work and war and women managed the home and children.

This individuation of families supported the capitalist dream of a free market, but the real cost was the entrapment of women who bore the brunt of 'invisible' labour. The reality of this rippled forth as a living nightmare inherited by daughters who were burdened by the impact of mothers who were unable to reach their full potential of financial, sensual and creative freedom, forever crippled and lost in the martyrdom of Motherhood.

Feminists did not fight for our rights or burn their bras to usher in the birth of burnout.

THERE IS a popular narrative that says, "Women can have and do it all" and whilst that perspective is nuanced, the fact remains that the 'all' in question is relative to each individual and everything has a season. With a strong support system in place to nurture and maintain one's vitality, then yes, absolutely, you can have it all… but too many women are frozen in survival mode just trying to make ends meet, living up to impossible standards and feeling completely inadequate when they compare themselves to others that promote ease and flow.

The reality is that behind the scenes, someone's ease and flow is most likely held by a supportive family, a healthy partnership, a nanny or au pair, education, intergenerational wealth and financial freedom, a regulated nervous system and a plethora of other privileges you can't see.

Whilst this is certainly beautiful for those women in a position to experience that level of support, it is not fair to assume that women can have and do it all, at least not all at once. This is especially important to understand if you are neurodivergent, have experienced poverty, c-PTSD from a traumatic upbringing or belong to a minority in general because it is not the same playing field. Yes, it's Motherhood but we all live on a different block!

The Importance of the Village

Historically, the village played a central role in supporting mothers through their initiation into motherhood. Women used to plan pregnancies with the seasons so that they would birth together in harmony with Nature.

Wise elders offered guidance, experienced mothers provided practical assistance and empathy and the community rallied to celebrate new life and share the joys and challenges of raising children. In short, the load was shared.

Intergenerational housing and communal support served multiple purposes. Firstly, it provided practical assistance with childcare, cooking and household chores, easing the burden on new parents and allowing the new mothers space to rest and recover.

Secondly, it offered emotional support, creating a safe space for mothers to express their fears, doubts and joys without judgment. Finally, it fostered a sense of belonging and connection, reinforcing that motherhood is not a solitary journey but a shared experience woven into the fabric of community life.

Children were modelled this symbiotic relationship of connection and grew up witnessing *rites of passage*, the changes of bodies, the natural ways of caring for and feeding an infant and the shifts in roles and responsibilities. Young girls grew up witnessing the natural ways of pregnancy, birth, breastfeeding and the sisterhood that rallied around to care for new mothers as they took care of their infants.

They knew that the health of the mother was related to the health of the village. Elders had an important role here, creating a cyclic loop of community connection. Children thus grew up with a deep sense of belonging and connection to the natural rhythms of life, perpetuating the intrinsic, symbiotic and balanced way of living as legacy.

TRANSITIONING to a village ethos in today's Western world and suburban sprawl requires innovation and adaptability. It begins with reimagining motherhood beyond the urban confines and fostering resilient communities, in person and online. Embracing diversity is essential in cultivating dynamic, innovative solutions to the challenges of modern Motherhood. Narrowing your social circle to only those who mirror your own experiences risks stagnation and limits growth for yourself and your children. True progress stems from collaboration and collective creativity, where we come together in common unity to support each other and the future generations that are birthed through us.

De-Urbansing Motherhood

Urbanisation can serve as a powerful metaphor for the disconnected nature of modern society and its impact on Motherhood. As cities expand and populations grow denser, the sense of community often diminishes with the suburban sprawl and fenced-off properties, replaced by anonymity and a lack of interpersonal connection. In this fast-paced urban environment, mothers can feel isolated, anxious and overwhelmed navigating the challenges of parenthood without the support networks that were once intrinsic to village life. It's no wonder postpartum depression affects many women. It is a symptom of a system out of alignment with *Natural Lore**.

The compartmentalisation of motherhood is manifold. In urban centres, time and resource-poor mothers often juggle multiple responsibilities, from employment obligations to childcare to household duties, with little time or space for meaningful interaction with other parents or community members.

---

* Lore references a body of knowledge, wisdom, tradition or ethos passed down (usually by way of oral storytelling) amongst members of a culture. In this context, Natural Lore speaks to the understanding of aligning and working with the rhythms, seasons, cycles and wisdom of nature.

This isolation can lead to feelings of loneliness, stress, guilt and burnout as mothers struggle to meet the demands of modern parenting without the traditional support systems that were once readily available. This workload is especially crippling for single mothers and is not natural.

Therefore, de-urbanising motherhood and reviving the village holds significant importance for healthy families and thriving communities. In a restored village, mothers are not alone on their journey; they have a network of friends, neighbours and mentors to lean on for advice, assistance and emotional support. Whether it's organising playgroups, sharing resources or simply lending a listening ear, the village provides a sense of solidarity and camaraderie essential for healthy families and thriving communities.

Effects on the Mother's Nervous System

The village's ecosystem is crucial to a mother's well-being, offering a shield against stress and fostering emotional resilience. By nurturing relationships within the community, mothers develop the capacity to rebound from life's challenges more readily, supported by a more balanced autonomic nervous system response. This environment of belonging and support also leads to improved mental health outcomes, reducing the risk of anxiety and depression. Ultimately, the village provides a nurturing space where mothers feel recognised, valued and emotionally supported, promoting relaxation and psychological rest, which flows on to the children.

The village provides a supportive setting where children learn to regulate their stress responses through co-regulation with caregivers, mitigating the impact of stress on their developing brains and bodies through social buffering. Moreover, interactions with diverse village members nurture essential social-emotional skills in children, such as empathy, communication and cooperation. These skills manifested in a well-integrated nervous system, enable children to adapt to social cues and cultivate healthy relationships.

Mothers and children who experience the nurturing support of the village are more likely to exhibit greater resilience in the face of adversity throughout their lives. This resilience stems from a well-regulated nervous system, strong social support networks and a deep-seated belief in their own capacity to overcome challenges. The village fosters the development of emotional intelligence in both mothers and children, leading to more fulfilling relationships, better mental health outcomes and greater overall life satisfaction. Individuals attuned to their own emotions and those of others are better equipped to navigate the complexities of modern life with grace and compassion.

Remedying the Disconnect: Simple Solutions

Prioritising the creation of supportive communities that honour the sacred journey of Motherhood helps cultivate a more resilient, compassionate and interconnected society for generations to come. So, how do we do this?

- Encouraging the formation of local support groups is paramount, providing platforms for mothers to come together, share experiences and offer mutual support. These gatherings, from casual coffee mornings to organised playdates and women's circles, serve as vital opportunities for women to connect, reviving ancient practices of sisterhood and nurturing bonds between mothers and children. If you can't join one, create one!
- Draw inspiration from traditional cultures where communal support thrives and reintroducing rituals like postpartum care and confinement can offer mothers much-needed rest and bonding time with their infants.
- Fostering intergenerational connections within the community further enriches the lives of young mothers and elderly members alike, promoting mentorship and mutual support through shared activities and storytelling sessions.
- Embracing workplace flexibility and promoting digital communities focused on motherhood also play integral roles in creating supportive environments for families, providing avenues for connection and resource-sharing.

As we reimagine Motherhood as a shared journey supported by the collective wisdom of the village, we channel our creativity to solutions and opportunities that help us grow strong and resilient together. In this way, we find common ground to walk gently forward to a future that strengthens and nurtures the physical, emotional and spiritual health and well-being of us all... in common unity.

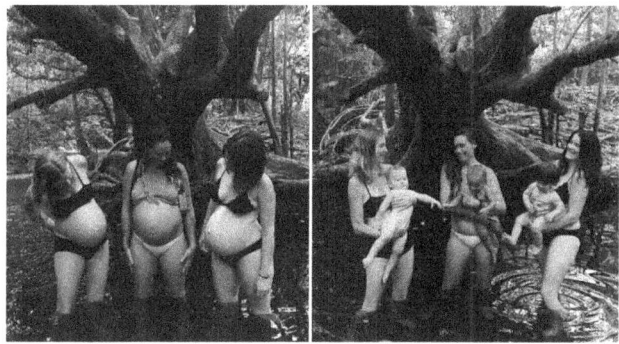

Photography by Jolene Reyes

PART VI SACRED BIRTH STORIES
MY JOURNEYS INTO THE PRIMAL WILD

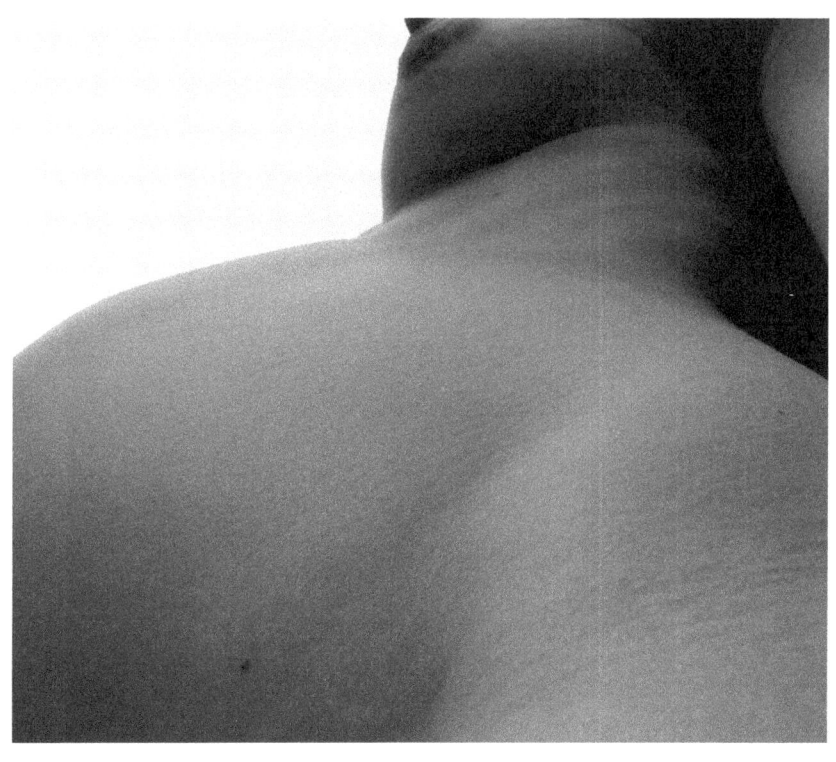

23

MY MAIDEN TO MOTHER JOURNEY
AURAURA'S BIRTH STORY

I finish writing this on the eve of Auraura's 7th Birthday. I was 18 when she spoke to me in my *dreaming*. She was a strong and gentle soul adamant about being birthed through me.

At first, I thought it was just my imagination running wild, creating stories. I knew from a young age that I was going to be a 'young mum'. I even knew I was going to be doing it alone at some stage. I had a vision of myself travelling the world with my little one.

When I first began to dialogue with this child, I felt a deep sense of responsibility that I couldn't really grasp at the time but I felt the power of what it would mean to become a mother.

Months passed and I started seeing a guy a few years older than me. I was completely infatuated in a young, lovestruck kind of way. He opened my eyes to a new world that changed my life forever and I knew it was possible to journey with him as parents.

This child in the ether stirred wildly, visiting me in my dreams and waking state. She was ready, but I wasn't. I kept tuning in to the realms of Spirit, of possibility and my potential children. I was seeking their names. Alorah and Zenith came through, but Alorah didn't resonate. Her energy grew stronger and stronger, and she was almost kind of pushy in her determination to be incarnated.

I pushed her away.

One day, I was driving to work and a bus pulled up beside me at the traffic lights. On the side, in massive letters, was written; AURORA. Alright, I said to myself laughing, "I get it!"

Around that time, I made a deal, more so out of frustration from this child's energy that was so full on. I said something to the effect of,

> "When you find your father, I will stop whatever I am doing at the time and I will commit to bringing you into the world. I trust that you know who he is and that you will make it known to me without a doubt."

I didn't feel her energy for another year after that. And that's when I met her dad. At a nightclub in Cairns called Freakquency. He was a VJ. I remember the first moment I saw him. He was surrounded by this blue auric light and he had really beautiful almond-shaped eyes, which caught my attention immediately and in an instant, I knew. I was completely infatuated and gave him my number but unfortunately, he had a girlfriend then.

About 5 months later, both single, we met up at the esplanade in Cairns. I was so nervous. On my break at work, I went to the local crystal shop and for some strange reason, spent my last $11 for the week on 5 crystals for him. I picked them at random and gifted them to him in a tree.

We started hanging out more regularly and one afternoon, we went to see his friends on the Atherton Tablelands. A woman working with energy named 'Auraura' (Which is where we got the spelling from, even though I didn't resonate with this woman or her work). That was the first time I had heard that name since dialoguing with this child's energy, and I took it as a subtle sign that my intuition was indeed correct.

3 months later, 2 days after the full moon, I knew instantly. My body was like clockwork and at first, there was the initial shock wave coursing through my body, followed by a rush of excitement,

"HOLY FUCK THIS IS ACTUALLY HAPPENING!"

It was just shy of 21. Happy birthday Donna, you're pregnant! I was in a bit of a predicament though as I had planned to set this beautiful moment to my partner that I loved him, but it never came to pass. And now this news. It was going to be a double whammy. I love you and I'm pregnant. The news wasn't completely welcomed. After what felt like a complete stab to the heart, I prepared my mental state to become a single mother. I rubbed by belly in bewilderment and said,

> "FUCK, This is happening. And I'm going to be doing it alone. it's ok, baby... just you and me, we'll get through this together, I promise."

I went to Townsville to visit my family and to celebrate my birthday. I was unsure of how to tell my mother. I took her out to lunch and shared the news. The response wasn't good either. In fact, without going into detail, the whole pregnancy was surrounded by negativity and some nasty energy. My father was quite supportive through it all, though he expressed that he wasn't exactly proud, but hey, what are you going to do? He often forwarded me messages from my mother and sister about what was being said behind my back.

My heart took a beating and I found myself consciously shielding my baby from this energy as much as I could.

"This is not my story," I would keep telling myself. "These are not my wounds."

I found solace through the support of my best friends. My partner overcame his initial fear of this new change and initiation into fatherhood. We pretty much spent the pregnancy getting to know each other. I was healthy, with no pregnancy symptoms except a few minor cravings.

Being a vegetarian was a challenge as I became borderline anemic, having to supplement with SPATONE, an iron-rich mineral drink from a well in Wales. I craved meat and went through a complete catharsis of belief structures I had cultivated. I began eating meat, which allowed me just to maintain healthy levels in my blood so as not to put me at high risk of hemorrhaging.

At 6 months, we moved into the *'Love Shack'*, a little humpy out the back of his grandparent's property. His father laid the first slab of cement when he discovered he would be a father to 24 years prior. It wasn't much, but it was free and we were happy. With our parents' help, we converted the run-down bush shack into a nice little home, ready to welcome our baby into the world.

I wanted to have a home birth, but the only midwife available was a guy that we felt was quite strange, so we decided the next best option was to give birth at the Mareeba Hospital in the midwife-led birthing centre.

My midwife, Gabrielle, was amazing in every way. I became a walking encyclopaedia during pregnancy, inhaling any information about birthing and baby development. Meeting Gabe inspired me to consider becoming a midwife in the future.

I was stung by a Scorpion when I was 7months pregnant. After a quick visit to the local hospital to check that everything was fine, my partner and I went along for our first antenatal class, which ended up being better than I had expected. Gabrielle was an absolute blessing as a midwife with such a vast array of wisdom to share.

At 40 weeks and 9 days, we visited Gabe for a check-up and to get some evening primrose oil to help things along as we had tried everything, sex, spicy food and walking up and down stairs.

I had two cervical sweeps and was 2cm dilated for 2 weeks. This baby was warm and snug inside my womb. That was a Saturday afternoon, and we discussed the protocol for me having to go to Cairns Hospital on Monday to discuss a potential induction. I was adamant that I was not being induced. Gabe stopped talking for a moment, cackled and said,

"AH! You're already there, girl!"

and then she ushered my partner over to have a look.

"You see that glow she has, that radiance coming from her eyes. You're in labour, my dear; I wouldn't be surprised if the baby comes tonight!"

She was right. At 3 am, I woke up with contractions. I was both scared and excited and rang the Mareeba hospital to let them know what was happening. My contractions were 10mins apart and regular. The midwife on duty told me to get some rest and call when they became closer together.

At 7 am in the morning, my contractions were 5 minutes apart. I called my mother (we had been on speaking terms since I was around 6months pregnant) to let her know that labour had started. She suggested we make our way to the hospital as we lived an easy half-hour drive away.

I don't remember much of the drive aside from me having my arse up on the dashboard, cradling the seat with my arms, absolutely tripping out on fractal geometries and what seemed to be this high-speed, inter-dimensional auditory transmission that I couldn't fully hear, but on some level could understand. I was completely high as a kite!

I think we made it to the hospital around mid-morning and were shown to the room where we would be staying. Unfortunately for us, it was out in the boondocks of the birthing centre, it wasn't even in the maternity ward, as strangely enough, they had 4 labouring women, unprecedented in this small rural hospital.

My contractions were still regular but had slowed down. We both chilled out in the room for a while and then I walked the grounds outside, hoping to allow labour to progress steadily. After lunch, the birthing suite became available and we moved in for the journey ahead. The room was dark and large enough to move around comfortably and I was lucky enough to have a private bathroom with a deep bathtub. I was very keen on waterbirthing.

Labour progressed slowly but surely. I jumped into the bath for a bit and had the most amazingly beautiful sound journey, where my breath and birth song sounded like a whalesong. I repeatedly sounded the words, "Oww" and elongated the vowels, which sounded so beautiful with the bathroom's acoustics.

I remember being outside my body, looking down at myself in this beautiful moment of fullness. When I returned to my body, I saw my other midwife, Jaya, with her eyes closed and a big smile in deep reverence for women in this sacred ritual and journey towards bringing life into the world. At that moment, I could feel how honoured she was to be a witness, as she would with all births before and after mine; she was there with Woman, completely present and grateful for the unfurling mystery.

The bath relaxed me into the process, but my contractions started to wane, and my flesh became wrinkled, so I began to walk the birth suite floor again and dance to the 'prog' music I had selected for my birth music.

One of my close friends arrived just after 4 pm and brought a delicious fruit salad. I remember the 3 of us, my partner and my best friend all gathered around the surgical bed eating fruit and laughing and then I would start to have a contraction and they would laugh even more. It was hilariously intense. My midwife came in to see how I was progressing. When she saw us, she let out her cackle and said,

> "Oh, you've got a while to go yet. You're still smiling. I'll come back and check on you later."

I made sure to keep my fluids up by drinking lots of water as that was drummed into my ear by multiple sources. The only problem for me was that every time I tried to go to the toilet, I would get a contraction and then I couldn't pee. This started to make things uncomfortable.

The contractions started to intensify at 2mins apart. I could feel that I was slowly approaching transition. Then my mother arrived. I don't remember much, but I do remember her energy ripping through the *birth field*, and subsequently, my contractions started to weaken. Gabe saw this and she told Mum to come outside for a bit.

A few hours later, at 6cm dilated, I had a bloody show. The smile was wiped from my face as soon as I started vomiting with contractions. It's not that I felt sick per se; it was more that my body was being overstimulated with intense sensations and the only way to respond was to throw up. I was glad we had fruit salad earlier, as the taste was still sweet and didn't burn like bile would have.

I remember having these moments with my partner holding my hands, going deep into my breath at the peak of the contraction and opening my eyes after the exhale only to see him looking completely blissed out and high on energy. Needless to say, I was a little pissed off! Haha.

I guess it must have been around 7 pm when my partner had a break for something to eat. I was in and out of the bath but couldn't get comfortable and the warm water seemed to slow the contractions. By this stage, I started to feel pressure in my pelvis and I squatted with an urge to bear down. Nothing.

I called, "Down baby, Down. Down baby, c'mon Down!"

I kept walking the floor and began to feel the stress in my calf muscles. My labour was creeping into the night and I noticed my friend had passed out asleep on the bean bag. Bless her for being up early and working all day only to come straight after work to support me. Gabrielle left me undisturbed and occasionally checked in to see how I was progressing. Apparently, all I kept saying to her was...

"From Maiden to Mother... Maiden to Mother"

That's how she knew that I was doing fine, completely committed to the process as it was happening. It was after midnight by this stage. I still hadn't peed and my legs were in excruciating pain. The pressure from my bladder and full bowels made it feel like I was having a full back labour.

I was becoming exhausted from being on my feet. Gabe suggested I get onto the birthing bed, which she positioned into a semi-reclined but upright position. Just being off my feet felt much better and the contractions started to build in intensity and frequency again.

I had passed transition and was 9cm dilated. I had no idea it would take so long to open a measly 3cm! Far out! I kept riding the peaks and valleys of my contractions but felt to get vocal. I started yelling. Not because I was in pain, but more because I could. I had seen this on TV and I was exhausted and frustrated. So I belted out a few loud "FUUUU-UUUUUUUKKKKKKKS!"

I was reminded to return to my breath and direct the sound down. A midwife by the name of Liz came in, looked me in the eye and said,

> "Right, this is what you're gonna do, you're gonna push like you need to do a big shit, ok? You can do this!"

It was probably about 1 am at this stage. My partner and friend each had a leg up near their shoulders, which provided counterpressure and leverage for me to begin to push. I was finally fully dilated.

Feeling so much pressure from not being able to pee, Gabe inserted a catheter and it honestly felt like 2L of water gushed out. It was such an amazing relief. Seriously, WOW! My contractions became even stronger and more rhythmic after that. Gabe directed me to push now that I felt how to do it. With a deep guttural grunt, I flexed my muscles and pushed them with each contraction. All of a sudden, Gabe said,

"Do you want to reach down and feel your baby's head?"

So I reached down and felt this soft, slimy bulge between my splayed legs. I thought it felt strange. Gabe continued to direct me to push. It seemed like another hour had passed. Gabe's tone of voice changed and she became more firm with her commands to push until we realised it wasn't the baby's head. My membranes hadn't broken yet, and I had bulging forewaters. I'll never forget Gabe's face when she said something like,

"Now, Donna, I know you said you wanted to have a completely natural birth with no interventions, but we have 3 options here. I can rupture the membranes myself, which will help things progress. We can wait for them to rupture; in that case, they will most likely burst and hit the wall, or your baby will be born in the caul."

She said all this with her hand placed on the membranes and her body slightly to the side with her head out of the way of possible fluid trajectory. It was pretty funny and her demeanour gave me a good giggle.

I was exhausted by this point, so I welcomed her to rupture the membranes. At once, I could feel a warm gush between my legs. A few minutes later, the contractions came back stronger and it finally felt like pushing was being productive.

I felt my baby's head start to crown, I reached down and could feel this warm, slimy sensation, a head full of hair! The intense sensations of contraction, expansion and stretching to allow the head to pass through started to creep in. Gabe called me to push, and rather than listen to her, I felt like riding through the contractions and allowing myself to rest for a moment.

Gabrielle continued calling me to push. I remember grunt yelling at her firmly,

"I'm letting it burn!"

This was in reference to my perineum, which felt like it was on fire and stretching at an exponential rate. My skin felt razor-sharp and thin and there was a fine line between expanding and splitting. The head was birthed, quickly followed by the rest of the body, into her papa's hands and placed directly onto my bare stomach.

I will never forget the first moment I looked at my first child… into pure, untainted consciousness. The most profoundly beautiful and surreal moment of my life. This little alien-like being had just found its way from my warm, watery womb into my arms.

Squinting, this precious little soul lifted her head and looked around the room. I didn't know newborns could do that! So strong and then the birth crawl started as she searched for the breast for a feed. 10 minutes later, the placenta was born and was such an amazing feeling of completion.

I decided to have a Lotus birth and Gabe found an old ice cream bucket in which to place the placenta. I am sure this was the first Lotus Birth for Gabe and the Mareeba Birth Centre.

I did it… after an intense initiation, I had made the transition from *Maiden to Mother.*

After about half an hour of bonding and imprinting time, Gabe asked what the baby's sex was. I reached my hand underneath the baby's bottom and said, "It's a girl!"

The last song that played just before she was born was 'Once Upon a Sea of Blissful Awareness' by Shpongle. We were allowed to bond for about an hour before it was time to move and clean up. A female doctor came in to do all the after-birth protocols. At first, I didn't want to put Auraura down, but my mum reassured me it was ok, that she was just getting measured.

My eyes became fixed on every movement like hawk eyes, sharp and focused. My body began tuning into every twitch and cry that Auraura made. I never expected the maternal instinct to hit me so strongly. It was a fiercely protective energy that, even after my baby was wrapped and asleep, I didn't want to leave her to go for a shower. Once again, my mother reassured me and told me to clean myself up. That was perhaps the funniest and most horrifying shower of my entire life.

Not only did my belly now resemble a massive jiggly tit since my belly button was still protruding but when I began washing all the blood from my legs, I reached down, and the expression on my face dropped.

"Oh no!" I said out loud and then I reached further. "Oh fuck... I hope all that goes back!"

They don't tell you about this part in antenatal classes. I passed a few large clots, which were pretty wild-looking, and then my mother came in with my change of clothes. I asked her to grab me a maternity pad I had purchased and put it in my hospital bag. Mum said, "Oh no, not those... here."

And then proceeded to hand me what I can only describe as an adult-sized nappy. I laughed at her, and then I realised she was actually serious. How the fuck do you put that on? was my first thought. Lucky mum had been so kind as to buy me a pair of granny knickers because my little bikini briefs would not be helpful.

I stayed in the hospital for 4 days recovering and making sure I felt confident with breastfeeding. One of the most intense afterbirth experiences for me was the lack of sleep and what I mean by this is that every time I went to fall into a deep sleep, I would snap out of it and stay awake. Even though Auraura was perfectly safe, warm and asleep- something kicked in where I would constantly check if she was still breathing. I was so exhausted in those first few days, It wasn't until we went home that I could finally rest. Little did I know that Auraura Freedom would test my wits in more ways than I ever thought imaginable.

24

THE BIRTH SHAMAN
MAIA LILY'S FREE BIRTH STORY

As I began to ripen in my pregnancy, I started to feel the disconnection between myself, baby and my husband ASM*. I felt so alone in the journey and how huge this transition would be. It seemed like his creative projects were more important than becoming a father for the first time as he was glued to the computer. I held my tongue for a while and just focused on preparing for my home birth.

At 38 weeks, I still didn't have a solid birth plan in place. I had tuned in with the baby and expressed how I wanted to freebirth at home. I felt completely clear and grounded on that journey, though I was very respectful of ASM as a first-time dad. I also mentioned that we could hire an independent midwife if he felt it would ease his anxiety about not having any medical professionals present. I met with a local midwife, but it still felt unnecessary. The money wasn't an issue; it was more of a feeling that I was meant to do this in complete trust.

My Blessing ceremony was beautiful. It was the same day the

---

* My second pregnancy and birth happened during my Saturn Return and was a very intense period of my life, newly married and separated within a year due to realising I was in a psychologically abusive relationship with someone who suffered from severe addiction and mental illness.

turquoise birth pool was delivered to the house by a local woman. The pool had held a safe passage for a few local homebirth babies, and I was honoured to be able to join in that circle. I had a beading ceremony and one to initiate 6yo Auraura into 'Big Sisterhood' we shared stories and food and my belly was adorned with henna by my friend Jilli from Henna Temple Cairns.

After the pool was positioned in the birthing room, the same room of conception we all gathered around and sang the space. ASM and I sat inside the pool, and everyone placed their hands around and started drumming. I felt the *birth field* start to open like a vortex.

In the following weeks, I was in the birth space every day, setting and preparing the space, singing, dancing, meditating, reading and sleeping. This would transcend the function of the room. It would be a portal to an enigmatic realm and I was the guardian of the gate. The sacred bridge. *The Birth Shaman.*

I still felt so alone on my journey that it surfaced much hurt. I felt abandoned and neglected by my husband in a time of need. Many trust issues surfaced, which became apparent as I was overdue.

With full intent, I kept anchoring the birthing space, singing, belly dancing and calling the baby in; I could feel the *birth field* vortex opening and swirling around my head over the tub. Everything was in place. Everything was ready.

I was walking every day, taking evening primrose internally and orally, having sex regularly for the prostaglandin to ripen the cervix and everything I could do to facilitate this birth.

I had organised two Doulas to be present for the birth, just to hold the outside energetic space. One was a local medicine woman with potent herbal wisdom; the other was a *Birth into Being* Practitioner. A few galactic alignments were leading up to the birth and one particular night during a 3-day cosmic alignment, we went into ceremony to naturally induce the baby with Blue/black Cohosh. I journeyed for the next 24 hours with the prepared tinctured, sitting on the grass in stillness, calling baby in.

I was having a lot of Braxton Hicks and was excited about potentially having a baby by morning, thinking it may be prodromal labour. Nothing. It was getting to the point where I was SO READY for the baby to come, but nothing was happening and I knew it was an energetic block. I tuned into baby and knew it was from 'Papa'. I had bitten my tongue for so long, felt like I was fulfilling my duty as a 'supportive wife,' trusting my husband's work, purpose and process, but I started to feel blocked.

So I approached ASM one night in his studio very firmly and expressed how I was feeling, how I felt that he wasn't connected, how this was such a sacred time and some of the most important work he will EVER do in his life as he prepares to become a father. I told him I needed his complete presence, that I could feel a blockage and it was coming from me not feeling safe or supported.

I was over his music video. Over it consuming his time and energy, over feeling like I was doing it alone, feeling like being a birthing mother was unimportant. That night, he came into the birth room for perhaps the first time with intention. It brought up a lot of my stuff. I expressed to him I didn't feel safe with him to be fully vulnerable in labour. I didn't trust him to be able to step up and support me, so I felt like I was holding on and I didn't want to feel that. I expressed how I was scared that if anything happened during labour, birth, postpartum, etc., I felt he wouldn't be able to help in an emergency as he didn't have his license (which I had requested he resolve years ago) and that this weighed on me.

All my insecurities came up at the birth's doorstep. I felt vulnerable. Although I felt like I had expressed myself honestly and respectfully, it wasn't received well and he stopped talking to me for a while. There were lots of tears and lots of healing. I share this as a reminder that any subconscious pain or unresolved tension that is not addressed and healed beforehand will show up at the doorstep of birth.

Labour

I continued to go for long walks every day and meet with my midwife. I found out that I was classed as 'high risk' because I had chosen to freebirth. This felt like an injustice and only gave rise to the birth activist in me.

Even though I had made a conscious choice to freebirth, I did not do so naively. I had a lot of systems in place in the event of an emergency.

The local Ambulance, as well as the Cairns one, were notified of my decision to give birth at home and were on standby in case of emergency with a request to take me to Mareeba Hospital unless the paramedics assessed the situation and would make the executive decision to transfer me to Cairns Base Hospital. I knew all the risks involved in birthing at home and still felt safe and secure in a deep internal knowing that everything was going to be fine.

I had no fear. I had given birth before. I knew my body. I knew the language of birth and was familiar with the space andwhat to do. It almost felt like I was guided to claim that choice, to be an example and show that it is possible to give birth safely and naturally at home.

I had been having contractions for a couple of days but had no physical sensation from the tightening, though they were visible. On the morning of 40+10 days, I went for a checkup with my midwife and requested a stretch and sweep, as I did with Auraura. After my appointment, I also saw a local Bowen Therapist who specialised in natural induction. I had a rest when I got home and went for another walk. I started cramping. By late afternoon, I had a show. The sweep and inductions worked. The ball was rolling, baby was coming but there were no contractions.

I felt like pre-labour was commencing and with the wisdom garnered from my last pregnancy, I decided to rest. Since I had decided to homebirth, my mother, mother-in-law and my close sister and birth support were requested to keep the space clear, which meant no visits unless asked, as I had begun to get overwhelmed with naturally playing 'hostess' to guests. Auraura was staying with her dad.

It was a challenge for me to express myself as I was just learning how to be assertive in my needs. I had a lovely meal that night and ASM and I decided to watch a bizarre foreign film. I wasn't interested in it and tried my hardest to stay awake. Eventually, I drifted off to sleep after midnight. I awoke around 4:30 am to the beginning of contractions. I got up, made some raisin toast and just sat in stillness, knowing all too well that I had crossed the threshold of the energetic doorway and into the *sacred rite of passage* of birth.

I emailed my father-in-law and let him know that labour had begun and that he would be hearing about the birth of his first grandchild soon. He did not come over from the USA with ASM's mother, so including him in this big life change felt right. I greeted the dawn in silence with a sense of purpose and clarity. I then started to fill the birth pool. ASM was still sleeping. Part of me didn't want to wake him.

I felt like I could labour and give birth on my own in silence and present him with his child as he woke up. It crossed my mind and I laughed to myself. Then, I felt that it would be disrespectful to do that.

Labour had started to set in and I began timing the contractions, which progressed from 20 min apart to 12, 7, 5 and 3. At around 6:30 am, I sent a message to Rachel, one of my best friends to start singing baby in. I'm unsure if it was sent, as it was a surreal experience trying to write a text message whilst in labour.

At approx 8:30am, after the birth pool was pretty much set up, I went into the room where Adam was still fast asleep. I laboured at the end of the bed, moaning deeply but gently. He didn't wake up. The contractions started to become more physically intense and sharp. I was coming into Transition. I called for Adam to wake up, telling him it was time.

I entered my birth space and laboured outside of the pool for a while as ASM fumbled around setting up the music. The contractions were intensifying and I got into the warm water. It was the middle of winter, so I kept a singlet on. This labour was different from my last as it was very 'in body'. It was physical and very clear, whereas with Aurura, I was hallucinating and being flooded with what I can only describe as a full DMT hit, in and out of this reality. Birth just happened to me, but this time I was more present.

With this birth, I could feel everything; I could feel the baby, the parameters of the room, the house, the town, the *birth field* and *womb grid* where I was connected to all other labouring mothers at the same time. I felt like I was communicating in a sacred, unspoken way. I could feel the enmeshment and fragility of life. I could feel mothers who had just lost their babies, lost their lives, mothers in both pain and bliss... it was all there. All apparent. I was connected to something much bigger than me. Pure, Sacred and whole.

At that moment, I became the *Birth Shaman,* travelling all dimensions to receive my child, to bring the baby through the sacred bridge safely. Guided by the wisdom of all Mothers who have walked and birthed before me. The web was crystalline and such a gift to experience and witness. In those moments of being in this Sacred portal, I received wisdom that I was requested to share with pregnant women to prepare them for the journey and to claim the Sacred birthing ways of Initiation. Deepening into *wombman.*

These precious moments of connection were interrupted by being offered frozen juice ice cubes and asked questions, which frustrated me immensely as I had expressed how I birthed and what space I needed to be held for me. Still, I had compassion for my husband as this was a new experience for him.

I remember when I realised, I needed someone else to hold space in the room. It wasn't that I needed help. I needed an anchor and although he did the best job he could in being supportive, I felt that my husband did not offer that grounded presence of strength and I needed him in the pool with me, applying counter pressure to my back. I needed someone else's hands to hold.

The birth supports were called and arrived soon after. When my medicine woman arrived, she asked me how I was doing. I looked up at her and she scanned me with her deep eyes, knowing it was all happening. She asked to check my bum (during labour, a reddish/purple line appears, which can help to measure dilation). I was in a full state of immobilisation as the adrenaline was surging through my body as my pelvis was opening to let baby's head pass through.

I reached down and told her I was crowning. I squeezed her hands through contractions. The labour was so internal and I was still, quiet and peaceful. Breathing with full presence and intention. I surrendered to birth and allowed my body to do the work and was simply breathing baby down. I kept repeating (not sure if out loud or internal) that,

> "We are ready to receive you, baby. You are so loved. We are here. We are ready."

A few moments later, I felt a familiar sensation. I reached down again to feel inside my vagina and realised what was happening. Unable to speak, I managed to pant, "Bulging... Forewaters".

I let my Doula know and kept breathing deeply. Consciously relaxing my jaw and throat, softening my mouth and relaxing into my body. I could feel the womb's natural *Fetal Ejection Response (FER)* intensely. It was such a profound sensation. Surreal!

My body and baby were doing all the work. I was a vessel...a conduit, the Sacred bridge. I remember going to my *dreaming* space and 'collecting' my child and walking the baby through a dimensional gateway. Claiming my role as *The Birth Shaman* and Mother.

Then, with a backup of intense surging pressure, the membranes burst with a BANG! and sent a ripple through the pool. Because I was in a wide-legged squat and so open, the impact felt like it rippled through my entire being. Like the universe had just ripped through me in multi-dimensional waves. A nanosecond after the rupture, I remember thinking, Holy fuck... here we go!

It was an intensely wild ride, feeling my baby descend upon its short journey down the birth canal. It felt like there was no reprieve between contractions. Baby wanted out. The FER was so strong it felt like the birth was happening way too fast and I had to summon all my strength to control my muscles to hold the baby so I wouldn't split myself open. I can not express enough how fast it was. it was Wild!

I felt the head begin to crown and reached down to clear away some mucous membranes. I could feel the baby's hair swaying in the water. My heart began to swell. I knew not to touch the baby's head during the crowning as it is very sensitive and can stimulate breathing. But it was just enough to have a very empowered primal sense of birthing as a process of action. The birth wasn't happening to me this time. I was actively engaged in physically facilitating the process. I fully claimed my role as Mother as I understood much more about this *Sacred rite of passage.*

Auraura arrived and quietly took her place beside me, stroking my head. The look of wonder and support in her eyes was so beautiful. She wanted to get in the pool, but I said no. So she stayed by me for a while, held my hand and whispered in my ears a few times. It was so precious that she was there to witness, and I knew what a gift this was to her, imprinting her for the future.

Baby's head was out and then I felt this ripple in the water; I asked Adam if he had moved because it was quite disorientating and an almost unnatural feeling of being rocked from the inside. I then realised I was feeling the 'corkscrew' turn that a baby makes to birth the body. I never pushed. I breathed deeply and let my baby and body do the work. It was one of the most profound experiences of my life.

ASM told me to lift myself up as I was squatting too low for the baby to come out. That was hard to move whilst you have a baby hanging in between your legs. The baby was birthed into its dad's hands and with a gentle grace in one fluid movement, I turned and he passed our child back under my leg into my arms. I held this new soul face down across my arms and slowly brought it to the surface. I noticed the first meconium passing just afterwards.

As I lifted the baby out of the water, lovingly stroking the back to stimulate breathing, there was this slight anticipation waiting for the first breath. It felt like it took ages and there it was, a gasp, a cough and a splutter. In less than an hour after transitioning at the end of my bed, I reached down and realised I had given birth to another daughter.

I didn't stay in the pool long and rested on a mattress I had prepared with towels and blankets. I was given 10 drops of Motherwort under my tongue and then rested with my new daughter upon my chest to initiate the birth crawl and her first feed from my breast. A rich and healthy placenta was passed within 10 minutes.

ASM, Auraura and I quietly sat together, gazing at this precious new family member. Such a beautiful moment. As with Auraura, I had a lotus birth. This time, I was more prepared for what that entailed. The grandmothers were welcomed into the space, followed by Auraura's dad and his pregnant partner. The room swelled with love as birth had come to completion.

The placenta was left to bleed out before we prepared it with salt and herbs wrapped in a special lotus bag that Rachel had made for me. Just before the placenta was transferred into the back, with my bare hands, I tore a 20c piece size of the placenta away from the mother's side. She flinched at that moment, which was pretty trippy. I tore this small portion of the placenta into 6 pieces, ingested one raw and froze the rest for later consumption during my hormonal transitions. It was such a primal and empowering act, as most mammals eat their afterbirth.

Although I felt strongly that my new daughter's name was "Ashama",

ASM said that it was too 'ghetto', whatever that means, and so we began calling in her new name. We liked Aaliyah, but there was a little girl who was not much older in our small town. Our second pick was Maia and then Iris. We settled for Maia.

Maia is a light, ethereal name with mystical overtones. In Greek legend, she was the fair-haired daughter of Atlas, who mothered Zeus's favourite illegitimate son, Hermes. To the Romans, Maia was the incarnation of the Earth mother and goddess of spring, after whom they named the month of May. Adam and I were married in May, so our marriage was to bring Maia into the world. I liked the idea of intoning my children with an positive attribute for their middle name. Clarity kept coming to me as that's what the birth represented to me. ASM suggested Lily, which means purity and was also his grandmother's favourite flower.

On day three, after the umbilical had fully dried out and was hanging by a thread causing irritations. We had a small naming ceremony in the lounge room with both grandmothers and big sister Auraura. ASM made a toast with a bottle of Anubis wine, her name was declared and I chewed the umbilical cord off with my teeth. It tasted like what I imagine jerky to taste like. So primal!

25

A VERY HOMELY FREEBIRTH
LUCAH'S BIRTH STORY

I met her in a dream. I think I was around 7months pregnant when I saw her face, she was wrapped in cloth in a carrier, with dark hair. She had a full face and little squinty eyes. She reminded me of an Inuit baby. It was the middle of a hot and humid North Queensland summer, the kind where the air is thick and the sun bites. Where you escape to freshwater creeks for solace or the shower if your pipes don't heat up.

My usual trick was to shower under the cold tap and then starfish naked under the fan! This was my first summer baby and in all honesty, the later part of the pregnancy sucked! It really took its toll on my body with low blood pressure and swollen, puffy ankles. I was craving ice intensely, crunching ice was so satisfying. I was addicted to the sensation of crunching it, literally cups of it. I started consuming more than what I could produce with my ice cube trays in the freezer and so I started buying bags of it. It was when a dear sister came over to henna my belly that she shared wisdom with respect to that being a sign of anemia. I had never heard of that. So off I go to get my bloods done, borderline again.

At 39 weeks pregnant I woke up in the morning to a sharp contraction that lasted about 30 seconds or more. I had been having *Braxton Hicks* for a couple of weeks, but this was a real contraction, the ones that feel like deep uterine cramping that start from the lower back and span around to the front like a hug that grips you from the inside, except it's not really warm and friendly. I was expecting to go over as I did with my 2 previous pregnancies, carrying to term at 40+10 and 40+11 weeks.

In the previous weeks, I had lost my mucous plug and then another at around 38 weeks. I knew my cervix was ripening and upon self-examination, I had started to dilate; as with my other births, I dilate quite a bit before I have a bloody show. Nothing much happened for the rest of the morning, perhaps another random long contraction around 9 am. I was feeling quite energized and started to get stuck into our domestic duties. You know that whole nesting thing!

I began gernying (high-pressure hose cleaning) the back deck from random leftover bits of playdough whilst my partner Jay was out mowing, and after he had a shower, we both sat down on the couch to relax. He turned and said, "Well, I'd say that was a rather productive day!"

We decided we would spend the rest of the day chilling out and watching movies. Just after lunchtime, I went to lie down with Maia in my room so I could have a nap, too. Something in me knew that I was in pre-labour, but I was not sure if I really wanted to be. Based on my last 'post date' pregnancies, I really wasn't expecting anything for a couple of weeks. At 39 weeks my dream of a spontaneous labour was about to become realised.

Laying in my bed, I texted my mother, who was 4hrs away, that I had had a contraction although nothing was regular yet and that I would know within the hour if it was Prodromal Labor and if she should get in the car to come up. The very loose plan was that she would come up for the birth, to photograph and to help with the girls. I say loose in the fact that I had become a little bit complacent with the fact that I was nearly full term; with this being my third baby and second free birth, I was still expecting to go post-term, in the peak of a very hot Australian summer.

Needless to say, I didn't get to have a nap with Maia. It had become apparent that I was in pre-labour as I had another contraction lying in bed with her. I couldn't rest my mind from the 'Am I in labour?' Chatter. Handy hint, it usually means you're in labour! I came out of the bedroom with a smile on my face, looked at my partner and said,

"So… I'm pretty sure we are going to have a Valentine's Day baby!"

Of all days. By this stage, it's after 1 pm. And we start setting up. My contractions are still irregular, but there is no mistaking them. I contacted Auraura's dad to bring her home, as she wanted to be there and witness the birth, just as she was for her sister Maia. Maia woke up super cranky as she does most days if it's in between sleep cycles. I was in no position to lay with her and settle her, so I tell her that Auraura will be home soon and that they can watch a movie. Bless her little heart, but she was incredibly whiney and clingy for the rest of the afternoon, obviously sensing the changes taking place, but not sure how to deal. That, and she was 2.5 years old.

Auraura arrived home and I greeted her out the front during contractions. They're about 20 minutes apart by that stage. We went inside and I settled the girls on the couch so that I could focus on setting up my birth space inside the *Womb Temple** while my partner tended to the birth pool.

We knew what was happening though there was no stress or need to rush. Even though we weren't really set up, we had everything we needed waiting. I decided to make popcorn for the girls. Jay was laughing at me and filming as I was having contractions near the stove. This would've been one of those risky jobs to palm off, especially with cranky Maia. Some jobs only mum can do! That day, it was popcorn!

I began to settle into the *Womb Temple* and then it becomes known that Auraura's father's car had broken down in the driveway and required a jumpstart. So Jay goes out to give him a hand. Auraura's other little sister comes cruising inside trying to find the other girls and as much as I loved her, it was not a good time for her to be in my space as the contractions had set in. It felt like so much was happening to take my focus out of the moment, like oh, don't mind me. I'm just having a baby over here! After they left, I felt myself settle into stillness.

I began to smudge the room and started singing her in. I felt to get my drum but for some reason, that didn't happen. I began to tune into

---

* The Womb Temple was a sacred space I had created in my home for women's circles, workshops and Red Tent gatherings.

my womb, to baby and then into my heart to send out my calling to all my sisters birthing at that moment, taking my place in the grand thread and tapestry of birth shamans, becoming the sacred bridge between worlds. I was now on birth's doorstep, about to cross the threshold.

Birth: Active labour begins

My hips began to sway and as I timed my contractions, I could feel myself dropping deeper into presence. Activating the spiral, moving my hips, breathing in slowly and becoming deeply anchored in my breath. I sensed that I was approaching transition. I loved my body and how she would speak to me, letting me know what I need to do in the moment to support her needs in opening the gateway.

I slowly got into the bath just on transition, listening to my body's wisdom, breathing into the oneness of all life; everything that exists in the peaceful presence of that perfect moment. I was still, calm and in deep surrender. There was a swirling of energy, a quickening and grounding and I became heavy in an ecstatic way. Everything was fluid and I was still, clam and centred, wading in the warm water.

I waited for her to tell me she was ready. I call to her in the ethers.

"I am ready now baby girl, Mama is ready now."

As the waves of intensity crashed over me and through my body, my focus was drawn to softening my jaw. I allowed my exhale to soften the body's response to tense up. I would breathe deeply and soften my whole body, opening wider. My body would spike with adrenaline and the familiar feeling of my pelvis opening. I could feel my baby descend into my pelvis, down into the birth canal. I continue to simply breathe and witness my child birth herself. Everything was so beautifully still and serene.

I could feel the pressure on my sacrum as my baby descended and without saying a word, Jay intuitively placed his big, warm hands on my lower back, applying counter pressure. My heart swelled with love for this man. He could read me. He's was just there, totally tuned in, totally with me in that moment. I kept thinking 'he's got me' and for the first time I felt myself fully surrender into the energy of the being held by the beloved. That feeling of being safe and so completely supported, a holy moment of union that was Sacred.

Then, like waves of piercing distraction, little Maia would rush in and out of the space. She needed mummy, and I simply could not meet her emotional needs with a baby sitting in my vagina. I offered the children to have free reign of the house, to use any sheets they could find to turn the whole house into a giant cubby, whatever, so long as they let me be for at least another 20 minutes. I reminded myself not to get cross with her as she was only 2.5 years old.

Rested in a wide-legged squat, I felt down and noticed that familiar feeling of bulging forewaters again. I prepared myself and gathered my strength for what I knew was to come. My mind was laser-focused and then POP! went the membranes! They weren't as intense as Maia's, though similar in the sense that the contractions picked up speed and intensity with no reprieve afterwards.

I felt her descend into the birth canal for a few beaths and then as she started to crown. It was all so quick and intense. I had to actively engage and used my pelvic muscles to hold her and allow my perineum to stretch. I had to command my energy to enable a moment to pause through the surging energy.

It was hard to breathe, the air was thick and humid and the heat from the warm water was almost unbearable. I shifted my face to find a cool breeze. I relaxed and softened as the contractions subsided, and then I could feel this 'slip' as if she went back up. I was met by another surge and she was right there, crowning again.

As I birthed her head, I could feel my bowels releasing a couple of nuggets into the pool. It's such an odd feeling, birthing and shitting at the same time, but there's so much pressure in that whole area it surprises me that many women don't know this about birth. That's the great thing about water births too, less mess!

You know, it's so hard to describe the fact that there was such a calmness inside the intensity. It was so quick but there was this internal serenity that took the edge off and it was all just so beautiful and blissful. So natural and totally normal.

One more contraction and our baby was birthed into her dada's hands. He passed her to me as I awkwardly turned around and then lifted my leg to claim our new daughter. Then the energy shifted and there is that moment...THAT holy moment, where the fabric of space and time felt so fragile, where everything, your whole world, could collapse in a silent second. Everything came to a halt! Breathe baby. BREATHE.

And this plump, purple fleshy being of love incarnate took its first breath. Life begins outside the womb. Life as a family begins. Life as a mother of 3 daughters. All the waiting, wishing and wondering collapsed with my relaxing shoulders as I cradled our daughter in my arms. I am reborn as a Mother. Bringing her to my chest for the first time, welcoming her home, Lucah.

In my heart, I thank the unspoken guild that I have now transitioned through and cheekily say, "Happy Valentines day baybee."

We share a moment together, just the 3 of us and as if perfectly timed, Auraura and Maia come into the *Womb Temple* to greet their new little sister. Auraura told me she felt the exact moment that Lucah was born and then brought Maia in.

I got out of the birth pool to birth the placenta. This was to monitor any blood loss, as I was borderline anemic, so there was a risk of hemorrhage. The placenta was birthed within 5 minutes, although part of the sac was still caught inside. I was unsure if the placenta had come away fully and if that was the reason the membranes were still inside. After about 5 minutes, I asked my partner to call my local independent midwife just to make sure. She gave me the all-clear to tug on it. An odd sensation but it released with another small gush of blood into the placenta bowl. We cut the umbilical cord about 4.5hrs later as it was summer and there were lots of flies around so it wasn't ideal for a full Lotus birth. Instead, I decided to print the placenta onto paper to create an artistic keepsake.[*]

We bonded for about an hour without any need to move. We were comfortable, safe and content at home. I looked at this beautiful and healthy baby girl and then realised she was exactly how I dreamed of

---

[*] Lucah's Placent Print video: https://bit.ly/placentaprint

her. So yes, to echo what Jay had said earlier, that was a rather productive day!

26

FROM A TO Z
ZENITH'S BIRTH STORY.

Flashback to about 16 years ago. We were 17 or 18 at the time. Jay and Donna, young and wildly in love since grade 9. I had booked a cute little cabin on Magnetic Island for a weekend getaway and we pretty much made love and explored Nelly Bay, which was newly under construction.

One night, we meandered the quiet streets until we walked to the wharf and found ourselves in a new subdivision with private little jetties. So we made our way down to one and sat by the water. Knowing us, we probably made out for a while and then stargazed. Life was so simple back then.

What I remember most about this moment is that we started dreaming about our life together. You see, at this stage, we had been together for 4 years, on and off again during high school dramas. We had shared many firsts and it seemed natural to our innocent hearts that we would settle down and have a family. So we started dreaming it in.

The most significant detail I remember amongst the inevitable nonsense was that we would have a blue house and a son which Jay named Quade. Apparently, that's what he was going to be named. I remember seeing this reality when I closed my eyes; it felt homely and safe. Unfortunately, our fate as lovers ended as I left my hometown, seeking soul-expanding experiences. We tried the long-distance thing, but it didn't last. It was time to grow, apart.

I landed in Melbourne and long story short, it was a pivotal moment in my life and significant in my timeline of self and spiritual development. I first moved there with 2 of my best friends, who returned to Queensland. So I was alone in a massive city, with no friends and no idea where I would live. I found a cute little place in Elwood on a beautiful treelined street, sharing with a guy named Damian and his long-haired German Shepherd. He was an eccentric vegan skateboarder who worked at Wendy's. A vegan, managing a huge ice cream franchise. The irony of this left me quite perplexed at the time. I pretty much kept to myself. I loved dogs, but the coating of dog hair over everything meant I didn't occupy the communal areas much and would often retreat to my room. During my stay in this shared house, I had some pretty intense and mystical experiences that blew my mind and fractured my experience of 'normal' reality.

One of those was feeling 2 *'star seeds'* come through my consciousness… my unborn children. A daughter named Allorah Freedom and a son named Zenith. These energies would visit me often, and I would have dreams about these children that I was to mother. As days passed, I realised that Allorah was Auraura and I had that confirmed by her fierce Spirit. She was to be my firstborn, and Zenith, well, he kinda took a back seat. I had never heard that name before or even knew what it meant. This was in 2004.

Ladies Before Gentlemen

I gave birth to Auraura when I was 21 and separated from her father around a year later. We gave it our best shot, though I knew deep down we were not meant to be and I always felt this longing in my heart to reconnect with the boy I gave my heart to, my first love, Jay. I moved back to Townsville to study for my art degree.

I tried to find him to reconnect and catch up. I knew he had a girlfriend and I was not interested in interfering with that, but he was my best friend and I wanted to see him. I called his parent's house, left messages, and contacted his sister and his partner. Access denied.

There was this intense energy in me that I wasn't sure if what I felt was real or limerence. I just knew I had to see him. If I could just look into those blue eyes, I would know in an instant. There was an insatiable yearning for reconnection. I just needed something, so I would know what the fuck was going on and why I couldn't stop thinking about him, whether I was just pining for the past or having premonitions of the future.

I lived in Townsville for 2 years and never saw him. I remember this intensity at one point when I skipped art school for the day and pleaded with the universe to tell me if this was meant to be or if my intuition was wrong, and I had to let go fully. When I got home, a red convertible was in the driveway across the road. It stood out because I'd never seen this car there and it looked totally out of place. The number plate read JAYO69. My whole body rushed. I was dumbfounded.

His sister ended up being my property manager and through our Facebook chat, I found out that things were pretty serious with Jay and his girlfriend, they would get married and there would be a baby soon. I figured he must be happy and in love. I found out he got married and my heart broke, but deep down, I was happy if they were. Our mutual best friend 'Jazza' would fill me in on what was happening in his world, that he had become a dad etc, but we were both pissed that we were never invited to the wedding.

I grieved deeply; this romanticised loss hit me hard, but I bunkered down and did the inner work until I was truly happy for him, his wife and his newborn son. It wasn't meant to be, it was all in my head. A story. A fantasy.

A few years later, I was married and gave birth to another beautiful daughter named Maia Lily. At the start of the pregnancy, I was convinced she was a boy because of her strong energy. I thought it was Zenith, but after a couple of months, I knew I was carrying a girl.

Jazza came to my wedding and told me that Jay was divorced. He was always filling me in on little snippets of what was happening, and I'm sure he was doing the same for Jay.

About a year after Maia was born, I was hit with the crippling awareness that I was in an abusive relationship dynamic and after many ignored red flags and traumatic events, mustered up the courage to walk away. It was a challenging time and during the last few months of trying everything I could not to face the reality of what was in front of me, Jay reached out via a Facebook message.

After 10 years of no communication. I was awestruck at the timing of all of this. WTF! Why now? When I was preparing to end my unhealthy marriage. WHY!?!

I met up with him, and our children played together. He had 2 sons, I had 2 daughters. I felt compelled to apologise and atone for my mistakes in our youthful relationship, owning up to the times when I didn't act very kindly and the impact my leaving had on him. He also apologised. Connecting and coming to peace with how everything played out felt for us both felt healing. I never told him my marriage was ending. I was super mindful only to give off platonic energy.

He told me he had a shotgun wedding because of the pregnancy. It's not what he wanted, but he was pressured to do the right thing. He told me that his ex-wife was now a lesbian and that things had become toxic towards the end of their marriage, with two sons.This all blew my mind. I had no idea. I thought he was happy. Clearly not. And I wasn't either, but I couldn't reveal any of that to him, though I wanted to.

I battled with myself about still being legally married, about having desires for another man. I spoke to my husband about all of this when I got home, completely transparent, raw and vulnerable because that was the respectful thing to do. I researched 'first love attachment bonds' because I thought maybe this was all psychological.

At the time, I didn't trust my own mind, which the by-product of the gaslighting and emotional abuse I was was experiencing. I tried one last time to revive my marriage, but the rose-coloured glasses had long been smashed and all I could see was toxicity. Our relationship was all based on an illusion and I was scared about my future on that path. I was terrified of mine and my children's safety. I was married for one year. Separating was one of the hardest and most liberating experiences of my life. Deep soul lessons were learned, and I did my best to navigate that with minimal damage for either party, especially my children.

So, as you can guess, Jay and I rekindled our love and magnetic connection with much hesitation and caution on my part. I was still healing, and I was guarded. It was only because we knew each other and had history that things progressed quicker than I would have been comfortable with had it been someone I had just met. We knew each other and now had a second chance not to take our connection for granted. Being in his presence made me feel calm and safe. It was so familiar yet so fresh and new.

In the initial days of reconnecting as friends, I remember going for a sunset walk. As we walked along the boardwalk, the deep pastel sunset and crashing waves below, I felt this sensation begin to swirl around me, and then I felt it. Our baby. Dancing in the ethers around us. The energy was so beautiful. I knew part of our journey together was to bring this soul through. I never told him that. It stayed with me inside my heart.

One day, as I went to see him at his house in Townsville, I was walking up the front stairs when I noticed something out of the corner of my eye. On the ground below, wedged into the corner of the house, underneath the stairs, was a blue box. Written on that blue box was the word Zenith. I froze.

"GET FUCKED!" was my initial reaction, "NO WAY!!!"

A wave of electric energy swept through my being, my palms went sweaty and my heart started racing. This was a sign!

It was like an 'ALL CLEAR' from Spirit that told me I had made the right choice, I was on the right path. I snapped a photograph and then carried on as if nothing significant had happened because I didn't know how to explain what that meant to me.

A year later, I gave birth to our first child, Lucah Belle. My third daughter and Jay's first. We spoke about having another child together and if that was the case, it needed to be by the time I was 33 because I didn't want to have any more babies after that. We had 5 children between us and it got to the point where we thought it probably wasn't a wise financial decision to bring another child into our family. I was so sure that she would be my last baby. I grieved so fully when I weaned her, soaking it all in. Well, I was wrong.

JAY KEPT TELLING me I needed a boy. I would always laugh in his face and tell him I didn't need any more children because, after a stage 2 prolapse with Lucah, I was scared to have another baby. I was worried about the toll it would take on my body. I was worried about our finances, raising 6 children. Most of all, I was seriously concerned about my mental health because the sleep deprivation and lack of support I experienced with Lucah nearly broke me.

I am actually surprised I survived those years without having a complete mental breakdown. I hid a lot of the damage under the strong woman persona, but honestly, those 2 years were the most intense of my life. In short, it was hellish and I feel like I made it through by the skin of my teeth.

I knew the moment Jay and I conceived again. The sex was out of this world amazing and up until that point, I had been cycling mapping, so we had been using the rhythm method for conception, which had worked perfectly for 18 months. Not this time. It was the tail end of my ovulation cycle, but I decided to take a morning after pill just in case. The next day, the condom fell off inside of me. We joked that he blew the lid off. Another emergency contraceptive. So yeah, they only work if you haven't yet ovulated.

To be honest, I think we both subconsciously knew there was another baby to come through. It makes sense. Even so, it was a shock to the system because we had both agreed that our blended family would be complete with Lucah. We had fully let go of entertaining the idea because of the impact on my health. Yet here we were, again.

When you have a large family, the news of another pregnancy is usually met with more shock than excitement. You start thinking about the impact this has on the world. Is it sustainable, etc.?

Yes, I have been blessed with fertility, but I also have a critical mind. I battled with whether this was a good idea. This battle between head and heart had me looking at termination. I knew I could never go through with it, but I felt like I *HAD* to look at all options to be a responsible adult.

11 years in, 3 spirals deep, I knew what Motherhood commanded from me, and I was so scared I just didn't have it in me. I was too weak to go another round. I was tired of being a strong woman. I was tired of being tired and I was shit scared of losing myself and becoming an

empty shell- completely deflated and defeated, sucked dry and crippled to the givings of Mother.

In all of those intense feelings, I kept tuning into my growing womb fruit and letting them know I was just processing my emotions and feelings, which were not entirely true, though they were valid.

Pregnancy

I knew I was pregnant with a boy. I knew Zenith was finally here. So I spoke to him. I journeyed in my *dreaming* and we made an agreement. I said the only way I could do this again was if he was super chill and a good sleeper and if his Spirit agreed, then I could do this. And so, we had a deal!

The pregnancy was so different to my previous three. I started showing early, and I didn't feel movements as early as I did with the girls at 12 weeks. I was initially worried and then put it down to an anterior placenta. I felt huge the whole way through. I knew he was a big boy, and he was incredibly strong. I dreamt of him and started to feel his very serious energy. I kept telling Jay that this bubba was super serious but totally chill. He didn't believe me.

We battled over names. We had a massive fight over the surname. Jay was adamant that his last name would be his and not hyphenated with mine. I didn't understand why it was only a big deal now when it never came up when I was pregnant with Lucah. This led me to have an unnecessary scan to confirm that I was indeed carrying a son to ease the tensions between us. It was the first time we had ever had an unresolvable conflict. The residual impact of this stayed with me for months.

During the scan at 24 weeks, I found out that I had a low-lying placenta. I wasn't too concerned because I knew there was plenty of stretching to do, and that would most likely bring the placenta up and away from the cervix. For peace of mind, I decided to have another scan at 36 weeks to double-check because I would be freebirthing at home again and wanted to ensure it was safe. This is the only form of assistance I had during my pregnancy.

Aside from the intense pain of symphysis pubis dysfunction (SPD), sciatica and a random bout of vertigo, my pregnancy was healthy and at 36 weeks, I had the all-clear that my placenta was sitting at 10cm away from my cervix. This gave me the relief I needed to begin to prepare myself emotionally for what would be my third free birth at home, only this time, it wouldn't be a waterbirth. My son was adamant that he wanted to be land-born, which felt beautiful to me, as my firstborn was also.

He had strong masculine energy, and I called him my little viking. I talked to him every day and felt him call me into action. He actually called me to get to work and do the things I had been putting off.

I launched my *Maiden to Mother* program with Sacred Pregnancy, Birth Shaman and Sacred Postpartum e-courses (I launched it on Mother's Day just before I found out I was pregnant) I launched Mystic Wombman Bootcamp and a few other mini e-courses as well as my 6month Wisdom Keeper Initiate Training and mentorship which was a huge birthing process on it's own. PHEW!

It's as though being pregnant brought with it a sense of urgency to do the things I had put off for years and suddenly, towards the end of the pregnancy, lots of intense emotion came up as I delved into some deeply profound shadow work, especially healing my father wound.

Jay and I were on the brink of separation and it was all so incredibly overwhelming. I started researching more names. In my heart, I knew, though I was still open to alternative ideas.

I liked Odin, Rune and Rumi, after my poetic ancestor. Jay was hooked on Ronny. I loved the name Quade from when we were teenagers, though I thought it was better as a middle name. What was interesting, though, is when I looked into the etymology behind Quade, I found that it was an Irish name meaning 'fourth-born', which in our circumstance was quite synchronistic, as he was the fourth child for us both. Mindblown! You simply can not plan these things!

I booked a 3-day retreat as a mental health holiday, so to speak, to give myself some much-needed 'me' time before the school holidays and to begin writing this book, *Maiden to Mother*.

My plan was to leave home on Thursday morning and be back Sunday, late afternoon. My plans were somewhat thwarted; I had organised little Lucah to be picked up and was just about to leave when I felt an odd sensation backing out of the driveway. I stopped halfway and then drove back up, only to discover a flat front tyre. I would have to wait and ask for help to change the tyre and get me back on the road. I arrived at my sweet little AirBnB cottage just after lunch and after bringing my stuff inside, made a cup of tea and sat down to begin writing.

The words poured out of me. I was living a dream, an actual creative writing retreat. Just me, copious amounts of tea, music, nature and my laptop and a super active baby! I was about 20,000 words in on Saturday, and during a pee break, I noticed bright red blood on the toilet paper. My heart began to race.

I was so convinced my little man was going to come early because I felt so huge and was having intense Braxton Hicks for weeks! I began to settle into the idea of potentially birthing my son on my own in the tub. I knew I could do it but didn't feel safe alone. I rang the hospital and spoke to a midwife to get some advice.

Considering I was so ripe, I decided to pack everything up just in case I went into labour that night. So I stopped writing and decided to soak in the spa, listen to music and drum in my son, who was still relatively nameless. Well, that's not entirely true; it was more that I hadn't claimed his name fully. And so, in a very vulnerable space, I began my *wombsong* practice to clear any emotional debris, connected with my son and sang him in.

Calling out his name. Zenith Quade. My whole body rushed with a surge of energy. I cried. Tears ran down my naked breasts and ripe womb. I cried so deeply. The wind outside swirled, majick was in the air. It had that mystical, electric feel like something BIG was happening. Nothing happened that night; there was no more spotting, so the next morning, I delved back into my writing before leaving at lunchtime and coming home around 3 pm feeling fresh and ready to give birth.

The days kept rolling by. Christmas came and went. Nothing happened, even though I was convinced he would come early. Then came New Year's. Still nothing. I knew Zenith was ROP* from mapping him, so during those last few weeks, I danced and did lots of movement exercises on my yoga ball to encourage optimal positioning because even

---

* ROP: Right Occiput Posterior

though posterior is a normal birth position, I was not keen on having back labour.

I drank lots of raspberry leaf tea and made delicious mousse made out of dates to help tone my uterus in preparation for birthing. The Braxton Hicks were insane this time around! During a summer heatwave, I was treated to an incredibly beautiful and deeply nourishing flower bath maternity photoshoot with my bestie, Chanel Baran.

Activating the Birth Spiral

At 39.5 weeks, I went into the rainforest one afternoon because I had a strong calling: I needed to record some birthing chants (check my YouTube channel) while I was ripe. It was the last thing that I needed to do. That day, I felt the birthing vortex open up, and Zenith told me he would come in 3 days. I knew he would be coming around lunchtime because of his name.

Everything was in place. All boxes ticked and it just became a waiting game. I was still undecided on what would happen during labour, mainly who would look after ALL the kids as it was school holidays. My Mother decided to come up to be on standby and I'm so grateful she did. She was the glue that held it all together.

I booked some acupuncture on Saturday to help relieve the unbearable tension in my hips and pelvis. The SPD was taking its toll on my energy levels because even walking was uncomfortable. The accupuncturist asked me if I wanted an induction and I accepted, knowing that it would only work if the baby was ready to come anyway. He told me if I hadn't gone into labour within 24hrs then I could come back, but I knew I'd be in labour on the Monday anyways, He confirmed I was very close to labour before he even put the needles in by checking my kidney/yin pulse.

That session was wild and incredibly profound. Shortly after, I recorded a video in the car to capture what I experienced. I lost part of my mucous plug that afternoon. Sunday came and the children were all wild as usual. We enjoyed a meal together and everyone said they were grateful to have NannaH there.

More mucous came away, my cervix was ripe. The baby had dropped, but he didn't feel fully engaged, so on Sunday night, I decided to try the *Miles Circuit* to encourage his head to engage. I went to bed afterwards and woke up at 4:30 am to a gentle internal POP! and then a gush. My waters broke.

I had never experienced that before. I couldn't move fast enough because of the SPD, so I called for Jay to grab me a towel quickly before I saturated the bed. After the gushing stopped, I got up and walked to the toilet. My knickers were flooded and with each step, more fluid would run down my leg into warm, sticky puddles on the floor. As this was all new to me, I took photos to document for my online courses. The amniotic fluid smelled like a sweet musk- almost like semen but different.

It was a gentle start to the morning. Nothing much happened after the initial waters breaking, except random gushes, enough to soak a couple of pads until 7:30ish, when I felt the first gentle surges of prodromal labour. I made some breakfast, had a cup of tea and went into the Womb Temple to start setting up, but Jay had already done it for me.

I added some essential oils to my diffuser and applied some to my belly. It took a while for any signs of true labour to establish. The surges were short and all over the pace. This was so different to my 3 previous experiences, where they would increase in intensity and decrease in intervals, progressively leading to a crescendo of wild feminine surges. These surges lasted about 10 seconds, enough for me to stop and focus on my breathing, but they were so weirdly sporadic, coming 20min, 5min and then 15min apart, then nothing for an hour. It was like a delicate and graceful dance. Gentle.

By 10:30 am, I was getting bored; I wondered if he was still in ROP because I had read posterior babies tend to engage later. I decided to do the Miles Circuit again to kickstart labour because I was ready to meet this little man. It was the peak of summer and school holidays. I was done with the cooking.

I got about 10 minutes into the Miles Circuit, and a MASSIVE surge coursed through my body. It was SO STRONG AND POWERFUL. It was like this pristine stillness, and then BAM! A deep dive into the intensity of birthing. From 0-100 in one second. That was it... game on, Donna!

This was to be my third free birth. I knew the language of birth. I was familiar with the territory. I am opened and welcomed into the Mystery.

The waves came thick and fast with little reprieve. I heard drumming and singing... like my ancestors were helping to open up the interdimensional gateway with their prayer songs and I was standing at the threshold, weeping because I had arrived, again. And my gosh, it was so fucking phenomenally beautiful. RAW. WILD. OPEN. All possibilities collide into the breath of the eternal now.

I retreated inwards as usual. Calm and focused, but this time, I was moaning and more vocal than my 2 other freebirths, which were relatively silent. I was on all fours, holding on to my big yoga ball; as the surges would rise, I would rise up on my haunches like a wild wolf mama and then surrender to my breath and the overwhelming sensations.

Oxytocin, Adrenaline... DMT. EVERYTHING FELT ALIVE. This familiar place I love and respected so much as the *Primal Wild*. This was my Sacred place where I am connected within the *womb grid* of all birthing Mothers, past, present and future. In this timeless realm I called to him,

"Mama's coming for you. Come on, Zenith...I've got you."

I felt my son descend into my birth canal; the surges were intense and fast as usual, my body doing the work. I simply focused on breathing, softening my jaw and crossing dimensions to bring my baby through safely. His head started crowning and I reached down to feel his warm, wet head full of hair. My heart burst. As his head emerged, I reached for my phone to see the time and managed to snap a pic... a birth selfie! As you do, well as I do.

After a couple of minutes, I realised he was stuck. He felt huge and I worked with my breath and the surges as usual, but he wasn't moving like he should have been. He WAS a big baby. I could feel every bit of him stretching and opening me. Jay started to worry a little bit and said, "ok, baby, it's time to come out now."

After what felt like another 5min, I reassured him it was ok. I was working on the inner realm, gathering my conscious brain and scanning for what to do and then, without even thinking, my body wisdom, maternal instinct and intuition kicked in to gear. I stuck my right leg out to a 90-degree angle, rocked forward a little to widen my pelvis and then slid my finger up inside to help free his shoulder. This was perhaps the most intensely primal experience I have ever had. In two more surges, he was out. Born into dada's hands... all 4.1kg at 11:38 am.

My 3rd free birth, safely at home. A peak experience of undisturbed birth and trusting my inner wisdom. Witnessed by his big sister and timekeeper, Auraura Freedom. From A to Z... Zenith Quade. Triple Capricorn. My little Viking had arrived safely. Our family was complete.

27

CHARLOTTE
MY ABORTION STORY

I was feeling quite lost and stuck in life, so I called my mum and asked for a tarot reading. The cards revealed that a catharsis was imminent, deeper than I had before. She said there would be messages around me of critical voices saying something like, "You can't do that...Who do you think you are?"

None of what she was saying resonated at the time, and my ego was like, yeah, yeah, I've gone deep before, but she kept saying this would be different. More intense. That I would completely break down. I decided to book a room on the beach in Palm Cove following an intense holiday season, with Jay working over eighty hours a week. It was just little old me holding the fort at home with four children.

I booked a massage from a local woman and was dropped off at her home, where I had a beautiful and magical experience in the late afternoon. As I lay on the table, the late afternoon sun trickled in through the rainforest canopy and something shifted in me. I felt strong birth vibes, and then the kookaburras started calling, *Googoogaga Googoogaga!*

I knew then that I was pregnant! I went back to our accommodation and there was an odd tension between Jay and I which was jarring, to say the least. The following morning as I was watching the rising dawn over the ocean, the kookaburras sang again. I took a pregnancy test that afternoon. The shock hit. FUCK!!! Decision time.

I pulled cards from my Sacred Rebels oracle deck. 5 cards revealed the initiation ahead. The last card I pulled was to symbolise a message from the baby. It was, life after death.

I booked a doctor's appointment and had my bloodwork taken. I booked in with the Cairns Sexual Health Clinic to see an *Options Nurse* to talk about my health and my choices of therapeutic termination. I then had more blood taken and booked in for a confirmation ultrasound as protocol. I was 90% sure of the path ahead and 10% not sure if this was the right thing to do. Was I playing god, was this meant to be or was my choice to say no meant to be? I came up sharp against my moral edges. Facing morality.

The truth is I knew my body couldn't handle another pregnancy without physical consequences that could impair my quality of life for the rest of my life.

"Put your health first...Why don't you think about yourself for once?... Never gamble with your health."

These words echoed in my ears, and the crossroads I stood at were big. Any direction I took would dramatically alter my life as a Mother of four or five children. I knew deep in my bones that terminating this pregnancy was the right thing to do for this child and myself. I am also incredibly maternal and love children and if I could have, I would have loved to have had another baby. It was to be the hardest and most excruciating decision I have ever made, but also the kindest and most loving. A paradox, I know.

Unless you are in those shoes, you will never understand the complexity of emotions that arise when you are deep in the trenches of motherhood and faced with what is the right thing to do, not the fantasy of the situation, but rather facing the stark reality of choices and their consequences on ALL levels.

As the pregnancy was in the very early stages, I was able to have a therapeutic abortion, which consisted of taking medication to stop the growth of the placenta and then pillules help to expel the 'products'. I asked Jay if he would put the first pill in my mouth. I wanted him to take some of the weight of this decision rather than being a casual bystander because I was so fucking pissed that I was in this position. Apparently, the choice and burden were mine. I was so exhausted.

He initially rejected the idea and said he couldn't do it. He didn't want to do it, which made me question whether he was rock solid in his decision. I needed him to be 100% sure as I needed to be myself because I did not want to move forward with regret. I wanted us to make this decision as a team. I did not want to carry guilt and shame on my back, let alone his. I watched the Roe vs Wade documentary. I read about abortions. I watched *#shoutyourabortion* series on YouTube. I looked at images on Google, preparing myself in all ways.

THE DOCTOR WAS warm and loving, like the 'options' nurse. All my tests returned positive to confirm the pregnancy and my bloodwork was sound. She gave me the pill, I gave it to my partner to place in my mouth. The doctor said she had never seen that done before and I expressed my reasoning. It was a quick shot onto my tongue, though all I could taste was the cigarette fumes on his fingertips and I remember being disgusted that this was my sensory experience. I hated his addictions. The process was unceremonious and real, so I swallowed, knowing that I was now the harbinger of death. I was once a woman who relished in her fertility, now terrified of it.

Later that day, around 6 hours later, I felt life leave my womb. The progesterone blockers had worked and I felt the familiar buzzing sensation of subtle energy turn to stillness. I knew that the veils between worlds had closed. My womb was now a tomb. I went to the shower and collapsed.

I had to call upon the wisdom and guidance of the Dark Mother to hold me as I birthed death and destruction with my own loving hands. The feeling was bittersweet and the mind chatter was relentless. What kind of a Mother kills her own child? What kind of a mother faces the morality of 'being' head-on, grounded like the trunk of a tree, ready to withstand the storm to come? Me.

And I did. I had to reach down into the very depths of my Soul to anchor to my truth as I navigated the depths of guilt and shame in a way that I had never ever conceived of bridging. It felt bigger than me. Like I was thrown into the deep end of a purulent concoction of vitriolic venom that many women before me were cast aside and we were all tarred by the same brush. Marked forever with silent scars.

I was now part of a statistic, 1 in 3 women, a sisterhood of women who made choices to terminate pregnancies for various reasons. A sisterhood of women who have been silenced and pushed into the shadows because it's too uncomfortable to talk about these things. Well, I will talk and brave the curses cast my way, for in my choice, I was gifted the power of '*NO*' and I now hold this medicine close to my heart.

Gathering things for my altar, I glanced over to see the title of a book on the shelf that read, 'The Choice'. 36 hours after taking the first pill, I could take the next four, two placed on either side of my mouth, between my gums and cheek. I was in a space of wanting to be present but also wanting to check out, to numb and not face the truth of the path ahead.

I went into the *Womb Temple* (a part of my home where I facilitated women's circles) and cleansed my space, preparing for the birth. Being cautious of the family dynamic, I wanted to time the journey so that I would be bleeding after midnight when I knew my small children would not wake. So, I decided to wait until 11:30 pm to take the pills. I prayed that I could walk this with grace and ease.

A part of me felt like I had to do things the hard way and make it as painful as possible, unmedicated. There was no way out but through and part of me wanted to feel the depths of it all, like I needed to punish myself and my body until I realised I was in enough anguish and pain. I didn't need to prove how strong I was, so I took the painkillers as directed. I started drumming my space and singing a song that came through intuitively.

> "*I never thought I'd be here, I'd be here, here I am.*
> *I never thought I'd be here, I'd be here, here I stand.*
> *It's a heavy pill to swallow, Bone Woman calls be through.*
>   *Bone Woman sings me true.*
> *Through my grief through my shame*

I will never be the same on the other side.
I never thought I'd be here, I'd be here, here I am.
I never thought it'd be clear to move through fear.
Here I stand.
It's a tough pill to swallow. Bone woman calls me through.
   Bone Woman sings me true.
Through my grief, through my shame,
I will never be the same on the other side.
I now know the power of no.
I bleed free, I let go."

I tuned in to the birthing vortex and connected with the Spirit of my baby. I said everything I needed to say to the effect of;

"I am sorry, please forgive me. I thank you, and I love you. You are loved and honoured; I will welcome you into my lineage as your ancestor, though I am not to be your Mother, for your journey is to not grow directly inside my womb. Thank you for all the gifts you have given me. I am forever blessed to have carried you for this long and as with all of my children, you are one of my greatest teachers. My life is forever changed by this journey with you. Thank you for walking this with me in Spirit and giving me the strength to let go, knowing this is the true path forward for us both."

With the pills sitting in the sides of my mouth, I sang my song and drummed for the 30 minutes that they had to be in my mouth.

HELD BY BONE WOMAN, I called in the blood. I lay on the couch in the *Womb Temple* space and knew I wanted to stay awake for the next hour or so until the miscarriage would begin. I decided to watch Vikings. After about 20 minutes, I started shaking and felt a cold chill. I knew this feeling. It's the familiar adrenalin spike at transition. I grabbed a blanket and focused on calming my mind. I decided to go into the lounge room, lie on the couch and get warm. 18 minutes into the second episode I watched, called *Baldur*, the character, Floki, says something to the effect of,

"...I can't change others, but I can change myself and I intend to stay this way... I owe it to the dead."

At that exact moment of him saying those last words, I felt the first gush of blood. I paused the show and looked at the clock. It was 1:11 am. And so I began to walk gently. I walked into the *Womb Temple*. Lit the birthing candle and cried the heaviest tears of my life so far.

" I never thought I'd be here, but here I am."

I took off my period-proof underwear with a maternity pad and I squatted over a metal singing bowl. I knew I needed to be with my blood. I would have been outside, but it was a stormy night, so it felt respectful to journey inside. In the exact same place I had freebirted my last two children, I birthed my 5-6week old fetus. The reality that this was a birth never eluded me and it was as Sacred as my four live births.

Alone. In the dark. I heard a mass fall into the bowl. I grabbed my phone to use as a torch and saw what looked to be the developing placenta. And then, if by pure majick and an answer to my prayers, there beside it, perfectly clean, with no blood, was what appeared to be a small glass wishing stone, only it wasn't. It was my baby. Contained perfectly inside the egg sac.

I blinked in disbelief and reached down to pick it up. It felt like firm jelly, and I gently scooped it up into my hand, placed it to my heart and wailed like I never have before. It was done. Completion. My grief was palpable.

The thunder rumbled in the distance and I entered a grieving Mother's realm. As primal and wild as birth, death holds the same space of beauty and reverence. And then I started to gush blood as I sat there in the deepest heartache, facing the brutal truth and profundity of the moment. In the stillness of the night, my womb cried its dark red river of blood and I was flooded with messages that came thick and fast through the ether. I grabbed a torch and looked at my dead baby.

I knew I had to confront mortality and morality head-on because this journey had pushed my moral compass into unchartered territory. As a map maker, I knew what the task ahead was, though I never fucking wanted any of it. I didn't want to be there but knew I had to be. As with all of my deepest initiations from Spirit, they have been through the darkest hours of insurmountable pain and I have been able to meet myself in the mess of my humanness to find the gift of accepting myself and my choices. And this was my choice.

I knew I had to confront the 'monster' within, but when I got there, in that moment, confronting the 'murderer,' as people say, all I could see was a woman who just wanted to do right by everyone, including herself. A Mother who thinks about the needs of everyone and herself because, as a mother of 4, you are confronted daily with the harsh realities of giving so much to your children because they deserve the best of you.

Partially formed, it looked like a little clear globular lizard with a tail. I could see no organs or limbs forming. I cried at how perfect creation was. I cried for the loss of potential and the gift of potential. I wailed at how beautifully sad this moment was. I grieved so deeply and viscerally that I held my foetus to my chest and sang to it before wrapping it in some tissue and placing it away for burial in the morning as my youngest had woken up and needed me.

Throughout the night, I had these maternal instincts to put a blanket on it because I didn't want it to get cold. As irrational as it was. It was a testament to how maternally connected I was and how brutal this decision was, even though it was the right decision to make.

The next morning, I prepared a place for burial and snipped a lock of my hair as a blanket so that part of me would be laid to rest, forever connected. As I filled the hole with dirt, I sang and cried, placed flowers onto the soil and sat, waiting for a sense of stillness and grace, which came gently.

I felt the Spirit of this baby circle around me, and it felt free. For the next 21 days, I would sit, sing and grieve, committing to the process of being with all my emotions. The Spirit of the child had revealed her name to me as Charlotte and when I went to look up the meaning of that name, I found that it was a derivative of Charles, which meant 'free man', and at that moment, I realised there is no truer freedom than death.

And I wept.

NOTES

2. Rotten Roots

1. Leinweber, J., Creedy, D.K., Rowe, H. and Gamble, J. (2017) 'Responses to birth trauma and prevalence of posttraumatic stress among Australian midwives', *Women and Birth*, 30(1), pp. 40–45. doi: 10.1016/j.wombi.2016.06.006. Epub 15 July 2016.
2. Dundes, L. (1987) 'The evolution of maternal birthing position', *American Journal of Public Health*, 77(5), pp. 636–641. https://doi.org/10.2105/AJPH.77.5.636 (Accessed: 9 December 2018).
3. Sims, J. M. (1885) *The Story of My Life*, ed. H. Marion-Sims, New York: D. Appleton & Company.
4. (1915) 'Twilight Sleep; is subject of a new investigation', *New York Times*, 31 January, Section MAGAZINE, p. 18.
5. (2012) 'Symphysiotomy Procedures: Discussion with Survivors of Symphysiotomy', *Oireachtas*, Wednesday, 13 June. Available at: [https://www.oireachtas.ie/en/debates/debate/joint_committee_on_justice_defence_and_equality/2012-06-13/2/#spk_60] (Accessed: 9 December 2018).

3. Ripples of Love

1. Tonetti-Vladimirova, E. (2006) 'The Limbic Imprint'. Archived 3 December 2013. Available at: https://web.archive.org/web/20131203141851/http://birthintobeing.com/index.php/articles/conscious-birth/limbic-imprint-eng (Accessed: December 8th 2018).
2. Elena Tonetti-Vladimirova (n.d.) *Birth Into Being*. Available at: https://birthintobeing.com (Accessed: 8 December 2018).
3. Centers for Disease Control and Prevention (CDC) (n.d.) *Epigenetics*. Available at: https://www.cdc.gov (Accessed: 8 December 2018).

6. Conception

1. Fitzpatrick, J. L., Willis, C., Devigili, A., Young, A., Carroll, M., Hunter, H. R. and Brison, D. R. (2020) 'Chemical signals from eggs facilitate cryptic female choice in humans', *Proceedings of the Royal Society B: Biological Sciences*, 287(1923), 20200805. Available at: https://pubmed.ncbi.nlm.nih.gov/32517615/ (Accessed: 16 December 2023).
2. Baerwald, A. R., Adams, G. P. and Pierson, R. A. (2003) 'A new model for ovarian follicular development during the human menstrual cycle', *Fertility and Sterility*, 80(1). Available at: https://www.sciencedirect.com/science/article/pii/S0015028203005442 (Accessed: 19 December 2023).

9. Birth Warrior

1. Moseley, L. (2013) *Why Things Hurt*, [video], TEDxAdelaide, Available at: https://www.youtube.com/watch?v=gwd-wLdIHjs (Accessed: February 2022)

2. Wikipedia (n.d.) 'Shadow (psychology)', *Wikipedia: The Free Encyclopedia*, Available at: https://en.wikipedia.org/wiki/Shadow_(psychology) (Accessed: 12 April 2021)

12. The Sacred Spiral

1. Australian Institute of Health and Welfare (AIHW) (2023) *Maternal deaths in Australia, Australia's mothers and babies: Web article*, Available at: https://www.aihw.gov.au/reports/mothers-babies/maternal-deaths-australia (Accessed: 2022)
2. Amnesty International (2011) *Facts on Induced Abortion Worldwide*, Available at: https://www.amnesty.org/en/what-we-do/sexual-and-reproductive-rights/abortion-facts/ (Accessed: 2023)
3. SUPPORT RESOURCES (maternal mental health, infant loss, disability and grief)
   PANDA.org.au
   mumspace.com.au
   grief.org.au
   beyondblue.org.au
   griefline.org.au
   lifeline.org.au
   rednosegriefandloss.org.au
   stillbirthfoundation.org.au
   sands.org.au
   tcfa.org.au
   nalag.org.au
   servicesaustralia.gov.au/what-help-there-when-child-dies?context=60101
   raisingchildren.net.au/grown-ups/services-support/services-families/disability-services-family
   acd.org.au/
   kindred.org.au

15. Mother

1. Wikipedia contributors (n.d.) *Elimination communication*, Available at: https://en.wikipedia.org/wiki/Elimination_communication (Accessed: 2023)
2. Dunstan Baby Language (n.d.) *Dunstan Baby Language,* Available at: https://dunstanbabies.com/ (Accessed: 2023)
3. Healthline (2023) *Dunstan Baby Language*, Available at: https://www.healthline.com/health/baby/dunstan-baby-language#takeaway (Accessed: 2023)

17. Womb Healing

1. Fritel, X., Varnoux, N., Zins, M., Breart, G. and Ringa, V. (2009) 'Symptomatic pelvic organ prolapse at midlife, quality of life, and risk factors', *Obstetrics & Gynecology*, 113(3), pp. 609–616.
2. Raju, T. N. K. and Singal, N. (2012) 'Optimal timing for clamping the umbilical cord after birth', *National Institutes of Health*, Available at: https://www.ncbi.nlm.nih.gov/pmc/articles/PMC3835342/ (Accessed: 2024)

18. The Art of Breastfeeding

1. To reference the article Stordal (2022) in Harvard style from the NCBI website, the format would be as follows:

    Harvard Style

    Stordal, B. (2022) 'Breastfeeding reduces the risk of breast cancer: A call for action in high-income countries with low rates of breastfeeding', National Institutes of Health, Available at: https://www.ncbi.nlm.nih.gov/pmc/articles/PMC9972148/ (Accessed: 2024).

19. Matresence

1. Orchard, E. R., Rutherford, H. J. V., Holmes, A. J. and Jamadar, S. D. (2022) 'Matrescence: lifetime impact of motherhood on cognition and the brain', *Neuroscience and Biobehavioral Reviews*, Available at: https://www.sciencedirect.com/science/article/pii/S1364661322003023 (Accessed: 2024)

VALUES LIST

Values List

- Ability
- Abundance
- Acceptance
- Accessibility
- Accomplishment
- Accountability
- Accuracy
- Achievement
- Acknowledgement
- Activeness
- Adaptability
- Adoration
- Adroitness
- Advancement
- Adventure
- Affection
- Affluence
- Aggressiveness
- Agility
- Alertness
- Altruism
- Amazement
- Ambition
- Amusement
- Anticipation
- Appreciation
- Approachability
- Approval
- Art
- Articulacy
- Artistry
- Assertiveness
- Assurance
- Attentiveness
- Attractiveness
- Audacity
- vailability
- Awareness
- Awe
- Balance
- Beauty
- Being the best
- Belonging
- Benevolence
- Bliss
- Boldness
- Bravery
- Brilliance
- Buoyancy
- Calmness
- Camaraderie
- Candor
- Capability
- Care
- Carefulness
- Celebrity
- Certainty
- Challenge
- Change
- Charity
- Charm
- Chastity
- Cheerfulness
- Clarity
- Cleanliness
- Clear-mindedness
- Cleverness
- Closeness
- Comfort
- Commitment
- Community
- Compassion
- Competence
- Competition
- Completion
- Composure
- Concentration
- Confidence
- Conformity
- Congruency
- Connection
- Consciousness
- Conservation
- Consistency
- Contentment
- Continuity
- Contribution
- Control
- Conviction
- Conviviality
- Coolness
- Cooperation
- Cordiality
- Correctness
- Country
- Courage
- Courtesy
- Craftiness
- Creativity
- Credibility
- Cunning
- Curiosity
- Daring
- Decisiveness
- Decorum
- Deference
- Delight
- Dependability
- Depth
- Desire
- Determination
- Devotion
- Devoutness
- Dexterity
- Dignity
- Diligence
- Direction
- Directness
- Discipline
- Discovery
- Discretion
- Diversity
- Dominance
- Dreaming
- Drive
- Duty
- Dynamism
- Eagerness
- Ease
- Economy
- Ecstasy
- Education
- Effectiveness
- Efficiency
- Elation
- Elegance
- Empathy
- Encouragement
- Endurance
- Energy
- Enjoyment
- Entertainment
- Enthusiasm
- Environmentalism
- Ethics
- Euphoria
- Excellence
- Excitement
- Exhilaration
- Expectancy
- Expediency
- Experience
- Expertise
- Exploration
- Expressiveness
- Extravagance
- Extroversion
- Exuberance
- Fairness
- Faith
- Fame
- Family
- Fascination
- Fashion
- Fearlessness
- Ferocity
- Fidelity
- Fierceness
- Financial Freedom
- Firmness
- Fitness
- Flexibility
- Flow
- Fluency
- Focus
- Fortitude
- Frankness
- Freedom
- Friendliness
- Friendship
- Frugality
- Fun
- Gallantry
- Generosity
- Gentility
- Giving
- Grace
- Gratitude
- Gregariousness
- Growth
- Guidance
- Happiness

Values List

Harmony	Liveliness	Polish	Support
Health	Logic	Popularity	Surprise
Heart	Longevity	Potency	Sustainability
Helpfulness	Love	Power	Symbiosis
Heroism	Loyalty	Practicality	Sympathy
Holiness	Majesty	Pragmatism	Synergy
Honesty	Making a difference	Precision	Teaching
Honor	Marriage	Preparedness	Teamwork
Hopefulness	Mastery	Saintliness	Temperance
Hospitality	Maturity	Sanguinity	Thankfulness
Humility	Meaning	Satisfaction	Thoroughness
Humor	Meekness	Science	Thoughtfulness
Hygiene	Mellowness	Security	Thrift
Imagination	Meticulousness	Self-control	Tidiness
Impact	Mindfulness	Selflessness	Timeliness
Impartiality	Modesty	Self-love	Traditionalism
Independence	Motivation	Self-reliance	Tranquility
Individuality	Mysteriousness	Self-respect	Transcendence
Industry	Nature	Sensitivity	Trust
Influence	Neatness	Sensuality	Trustworthiness
Ingenuity	Nerve	Serenity	Truth
Inquisitiveness	Nonconformity	Service	Understanding
Insightfulness	Obedience	Sexiness	Uniqueness
Inspiration	Open-mindedness	Sexuality	Unity
Integrity	Openness	Sharing	Usefulness
Intellect	Optimism	Shrewdness	Utility
Intelligence	Order	Significance	Valor
Intensity	Organization	Silence	Variety
Intimacy	Originality	Silliness	Victory
Intrepidness	Outdoors	Simplicity	Vigor
Introspection	Outlandishness	Sincerity	Virtue
Introversion	Outrageousness	Skillfulness	Vision
Intuition	Partnership	Solidarity	Vitality
Intuitiveness	Patience	Solitude	Vivacity
Inventiveness	Passion	Sophistication	Volunteering
Investing	Peace	Soundness	Warm-heartedness
Involvemen	Perceptiveness	Speed	Warmth
Joy	Perfection	Spirit	Watchfulness
Judiciousness	Perkiness	Spirituality	Wealth
Justice	Perseverance	Spontaneity	Willfulness
Keenness	Persistence	Spunk	Willingness
Kindness	Persuasiveness	Stability	Winning
Knowledge	Philanthropy	Status	Wisdom
Leadership	Piety	Stealth	Wittiness
Learning	Playfulness	Stillness	Wonder
Liberation	Pleasantness	Strength	Worthiness
Liberty	Pleasure	Structure	Youthfulness
Lightness	Poise	Success	Zeal

ABOUT THE AUTHOR

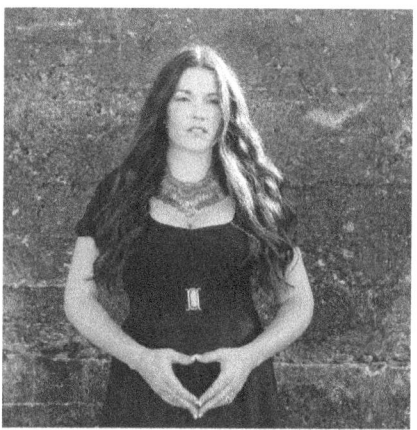

www.DonnaRaymond.com.au

Donna Raymond is a catalyst for transformation, creative expression and embodied wisdom. With 15 years experience as a visionary speaker, intuitive mentor, transformational leader, spiritual consultant and ceremonialist, she has devoted her life to guiding women through their initiation processes and sacred rites of passage in both life and business. In 2022, she was honoured as a finalist for the *Cairns Business Women's Club Sole Entrepreneur of the Year*, recognising her significant impact on women in the local community.

Nestled in the tranquil beauty of Far North Queensland, Australia, Donna is renowned for her ability to create potent transformative experiences through sacred circles, ceremonies, retreats, online courses, group programs, keynote speaking and private 1:1 bespoke mentoring. Her uniquely intuitive and experiential approach masterfully blends the practical with the mystical, inspiring and empowering women to break through limitations and cultivate resilience. She encourages women at all stages of life to embrace sensuality and playfulness while gaining unwavering clarity and confidence in their ability to transform challenges into opportunities for growth and empowerment.

Through the *Wise Wombman Wisdom School*, Donna empowered thousands of women globally by crafting safe, transformational spaces that nurtured personal development, deep healing, creativity, sisterhood and a profound connection to nature and the mystical world. After a decade of service, she closed the school to focus on personalised mentoring and continuing to inspire and guide women through other avenues.

Her latest book, *Maiden to Mother*, offers an intimate exploration of her journey as a free-birthing mother of four, providing profound insights into the sacred initiation of motherhood. This book not only reflects her legacy as a mother; it embodies the essence of her work, guiding women through transformative journeys of self-discovery and reminding them to access the wisdom within.

Whether navigating catharsis or inspiring creative expansion and innovation, Donna's mission is to help women unlock their inner wisdom, step into their authentic power and cultivate deeply fulfilling lives brimming with playfulness, purpose and wonder.

facebook.com/DonnaRaymondWiseWombman
instagram.com/_donnaraymond_
tiktok.com/@donna.raymond
youtube.com/@DRaymond

www.ingramcontent.com/pod-product-compliance
Lightning Source LLC
Chambersburg PA
CBHW062045290426
44109CB00027B/2733